MW00657658

Sasha-

Keep fighting the good fight! The path to achieving your goals is one that's up + down. It's all about resilience!

♡, Beth

Praise for *The Effortless Perfection Myth*

"A much-needed roadmap to challenging the damaging and insidious power of the Effortless Perfection ideal. A phenomenal resource for girls, parents, and schools grappling with problems they haven't had the language to describe until now."

-Soraya Chemaly, acclaimed author of *Rage Becomes Her*,
a *Washington Post* and *NPR* "Best Book" Selection

"*The Effortless Perfection Myth* explores and explains unsustainable cultural norms, including resonant stories of young women who are excelling without appearing to break a sweat, pleasing others at the expense of self-care, kneeling at the altar of evolving social demands, and subordinating dreams for community-prescribed expectations. Caralena delivers an invaluable toolkit, offering insights to help navigate and negotiate these dynamics of an eventful college life along with constructive behaviors to build confidence and comfort in one's own agency."

-Lisa Borders, co-founder & CEO of Golden Glow Media
and former president of the WNBA

"Our foundation does a great deal of work focused on perfectionism, social media, and the myths we portray for others in our online lives and even our day-to-day lives. Caralena describes these different lives we project as 'perfect,' and gives us a clear strategy for leaving those toxic tendencies behind and moving toward a more authentic mode of being. I highly recommend this book for all young adults, especially for anyone struggling with perfectionism or mental illness, or even those who just feel lost on their current path."

-Carli Bushoven, executive director of the Madison Holleran Foundation and
Active Minds mental health speaker

"A raw and realistic portrayal of the challenges facing the next generation of women in the digital era of social media pressures, this book is the ultimate survival guide for any young woman entering high school or college seeking self-empowerment. Caralena is a brilliant storyteller and captures the truth and struggles of what it means to be a woman in the modern age—complex, inspiring, and full of hope."

-Larissa May, founder of #HalfTheStory

"Caralena Peterson is like an older sister who's been in the trenches at college and has returned to report what you need to hear. With compellingly personal, frank anecdotes and tremendous compassion and empathy, she demonstrates the many ways that an idealization of Effortless Perfection can damage good people—and offers a roadmap for a way out."

-Leora Tanenbaum, author of
I Am Not a Slut: Slut-Shaming in the Age of the Internet

"Forget dorm decor: *The Effortless Perfection Myth* provides the tools and insights young women actually need to combat a daily deluge of toxic messages that make the already difficult process of growing up even harder. With heartfelt candor (and loads of research), Peterson helps readers discover why striving for 'perfection' is a waste of time and helps them learn to look inward—instead of outward—to discover the power of rejecting the Myth."

-Julie Scelfo, journalist, former *New York Times* staff writer,
and author of *The Women Who Made New York*

"While women have grown stronger, as *The Effortless Perfection Myth* so well documents through stories and statistics, internally they are struggling. Today's young women are caught between a generation of women who measured their value on being a societally sanctioned 'good' woman and a generation of feminists who upped the ante on what was possible. As Peterson shares her personal truths, she inspires each reader to find her own."

-Amy Richards, co-author of *Manifesta* and *Grassroots*, producer of Emmy
nominated series WOMAN for *Viceland,* and co-founder of Third Wave Fund

"This volume is a rare gift. Demystifying the Myth of Effortless Perfection is the first offering. Analyzing its impact and cultural origins is a priceless second. The third and rarest gift structures the book's five sections: concrete tools for young women and their allies to control their identities. Bravo!"

-Jean O'Barr, PhD, founding director of the Duke Women's Studies Program
(1983-2000)

"*The Effortless Perfection Myth* offers a deep dive into the phenomenon that is so destructive to women's minds, bodies, and spirits. Peterson dissects the many strands of Effortless Perfection and offers useful strategies to challenge it in service of a more integrated, confident, and authentic self."

-Donna Lisker, PhD, chief of staff for Brown University's Office of Senior Vice President for Advancement and former member of the Duke University Women's Initiative Steering Committee by which the term "Effortless Perfection" was coined

"Anyone hoping to understand the lived experiences of young women today, whether you are a parent, educator, or mental health clinician, should read *The Effortless Perfection Myth*. Peterson weaves in powerful narratives from women from a range of backgrounds, emphasizing intersectionality and stressors especially relevant to women in college today. This text should be required reading."

-Sarah E. Domoff, PhD, clinical child psychologist and associate professor of psychology at Central Michigan University

"Peterson has put tremendous effort into analyzing Effortless Perfection from all angles, affording readers an opportunity to explore and reflect on this troubling facet of our society that is not often given a spotlight."

-Nancy Redd, *New York Times* bestselling author of *BODY DRAMA*

"Caralena Peterson's book is a must-read for young women who want to do big things. Her book helps untangle the societal forces that hold young women back and burn them out as they try to be everything they think is expected of them. She offers a new path that is healthier and more fulfilling, and that ultimately will allow women to rise to power and influence—not as who they think society wants them to be, but as their true, authentic selves. And while the book is written from the young woman's perspective, it resonates deeply for women of all ages."

-Susannah Wellford, CEO and founder of Running Start

"I have been working with teenage girls and parents for over 20 years and have never read a book like this one. It puts you right in the mind of a young woman and the pressure she faces to be perfect in everything she does. Caralena is able to get right to the heart of the matter and offer solutions. Through personal stories, both hers and others' she has interviewed, Caralena shines a bright light on what females face in today's world. This is a must-read for teenage girls, young women heading off to college, and parents who want to stay a step ahead of their girls."

-Patsy Mangas, founder of She Rocks the World

"Peterson's work is timely, honest, and well researched—a must-read for young women and their parents. Peterson blasts outdated and often deeply ingrained views about women's self-esteem, confidence, and assertiveness, sharply admonishing those seeking the unattainable. Reading her work is akin to having that really great talk with your smartest group of girlfriends. Women's empowerment at its best."

-Peggy Tighe, JD, former president of Women in Government Relations

"Caralena Peterson's book is a much-needed voice for our society's young women who pressure themselves to appear perfect and for those who wish to support them. The perfectionism trap can be tremendously damaging, and it is fueled by the pervasiveness of social media in this generation. Peterson has broken through the dominant narrative to reveal essential truths that can become lost in the pursuit of success. I wish I had read a book like this earlier in life, and will urge every young woman I know to read this book and internalize its important messages to heart."

-Maria Leonard Olsen, host of "Becoming Your Best Version" podcast and WPFW-FM 98.3 "Inside Out Collective" radio show co-host

The Effortless Perfection Myth

Debunking the Myth and Revealing the Path to Empowerment for Today's College Women

Caralena Peterson

Author photograph by Chelsea Pieroni
Illustrations by Alex Lark

Paperback ISBN: 978-1-63337-583-3
Hardback ISBN: 978-1-63337-667-0
E-Book ISBN: 978-1-63337-585-7

Printed in the United States of America
1 3 5 7 9 10 8 6 4 2

Dedicated to Gary Glass

I hope one day to impact even half the number of people you have.
Thank you for truly life-changing mentorship.

Table of Contents

Effortless Perfection:

"The expectation that one would be smart, accomplished, fit, beautiful, and popular, and that all this would happen without visible effort."

—Duke University Women's Initiative Report, 2003

"Someday, sometime, you will be sitting somewhere. A berm overlooking a pond in Vermont. The lip of the Grand Canyon at sunset. A seat on the subway. And something bad will have happened: You will have lost someone you loved, or failed at something at which you badly wanted to succeed. And sitting there, you will fall into the center of yourself. You will look for some core to sustain you. And if you have been perfect all your life and have managed to meet all the expectations of your family, your friends, your community, your society, chances are excellent that there will be a black hole where that core ought to be. I don't want anyone I know to take that terrible chance. And the only way to avoid it is to listen to that small voice inside you that tells you to make mischief, to have fun, to be contrarian, to go another way."

—Anna Quindlen, Pulitzer-Winning *New York Times* Columnist and Author

Preface

EXPERIENCING THE PLEASURES as well as the pains of undergraduate life at Duke University gave me valuable insight for this book. By the time I arrived for my freshman year in 2010, the term "Effortless Perfection" had been a widely circulated phrase on campus for almost a decade. Naming the phenomenon, however, hadn't done much to alter a college culture that places immense pressure on its students to excel in all categories and to do so with a never-faltering front of confident ease.

Duke has a reputation for being an intense university where the many extremes of today's "youth" culture have been compounded into the "work hard, play hard" mentality that comes along with Effortless Perfection. This mentality, despite being somewhat proudly celebrated and propagated by students, comes with a disconcerting underbelly of undue pressures. When left unchecked, as is often the case, these pressures manifest themselves as serious social problems, including stress, anxiety, loneliness, binge drinking, eating disorders, unauthentic and unhealthy sexual expression, and depression.

I certainly wasn't one to dodge the bullet on most of these. Throughout all my many joys and excitements as an undergrad, several of these issues remained a constant undercurrent. I was always struggling with two or more at a time. I might as well have been a case study for the effects of the Effortless Perfection Myth. After all, I was already attending Duke, where the term originated, and thus the perfect backdrop for studying and understanding the Myth. Mix in the outlook of an eager but naive teen and the temperament of a people-pleasing "good girl" I brought with me to campus, and my fate was basically sealed.

What kept me afloat was my strong desire to analyze what was happening to me and why. The further I pushed into the space existing behind the gilded front of Effortless Perfection, the more I found it wasn't just me—so many of the people who looked like they had everything all put together, their lives completely figured out, were struggling just the same or even worse. This issue needed serious attention.

Effortless Perfection had created an environment wherein each person who inevitably struggled was sure to feel like the only one. Feeling isolated, each would grow fearful of being exposed as someone who "couldn't keep up" or who stood out as "broken" in comparison to the rest of a presumably flawless student body. So they would conclude that the only way to deal with problems was to do it alone. Thus the consequences of their struggles became much more extreme and much more harmful.

I wanted to believe it didn't have to be this way. I found myself drawn to the few spaces on campus where authentic discussions were happening. I found myself sharing some of my own vulnerabilities as a way of making others feel more comfortable with sharing their own, and I could see the relief in their eyes as they finally let what was happening in their inner worlds be known. I looked to grow the discourse via mentoring programs, student-led initiatives, an opinion column in my school newspaper, and even just spontaneous conversation. I declared a women's studies major because I could see my female peers being hit especially hard and wanted to know why. I could feel the puzzle of Effortless Perfection being pieced together in my head as I went, and could see it being exposed as the Myth I now know it to be.

Over time I discovered that the insights I was gleaning along this journey were incredible privileges to possess—even though many had required intense personal struggle to acquire—because they blessed me with the ability to mentor others experiencing similar hardships and to help them not feel so alone. Knowing what a person in the midst of struggle needs is difficult unless you yourself have been there too, as you can only *fully* empathize with someone to the extent that you have personally felt what that person is feeling.

Most times, those who are hurting don't want to be "fixed" or told what to do. They just want proof that it is possible to go through these jolting realizations about the nature of our unpredictable and sometimes overwhelming world and come out the other side. They want someone to be with them, to feel with them, to understand. They want someone who can say, "Me too, I've been there." *This book is meant to be a compilation of all that I have to give in this way.* It is the book I wish I had been able to read before entering college, to gain an understanding of what I would encounter on campus as an undergrad.

Although my personal experience is limited to four and a half years at one school, the issues I address are universal. Effortless Perfection is definitely not just a Duke thing; it plagues college students in any high-intensity/high-expectation environment. Young women all across the country have come to use this term when describing the cultural climate on their campuses, which is why I made sure to include narratives and commentary from my female peers at a range of schools, including Colgate, Georgetown, High Point, New York University, Northwestern, Pitzer, University of Alabama, University of California–San Diego, University of Maryland, University of Pennsylvania, Vanderbilt, and Virginia Tech (all have been given pseudonyms to protect their privacy). What I write in this book is meant to be relevant and useful to today's generation of college students as a whole.

I have done extensive research into the issues of race, sexuality, and socioeconomic status, and invested much of my time as an undergrad in spaces and programs meant for navigating and embracing diversity. Yet I am only one person, so I believe it is important to note that I have identity markers that have both allowed me and forced me to experience college through particular lenses. Still, I have collected research from a variety of sources to cover the concept of Effortless Perfection as fully and effectively as possible. My interviewees represent a diversity of races, sexualities, and socioeconomic statuses. I fervently believe there is something in here for everyone, especially because I have put great effort into making this book as intersectional and inclusive as I know how.

As you read, you will notice I say "we" and "our" a great deal, identifying myself with the collegiate women whose stories I'm telling. I do so because I've sensed that many parents, professors, university administrators, and clinicians are in search of frank dialogue about what is happening on undergraduate campuses today. This book provides the straightforward answers they are looking for while giving them the feeling they are being let in on a secret. It also discusses these topics in a way that still feels accessible to female undergrads. A parent might read a chapter and think, *my daughter needs to read this!* Alternativiely, a female undergrad might just pick up the text of her own accord.

The goal is to keep the book feeling accessible for both audiences—those experiencing these struggles in the here and now and all those looking to support them. To further dialogue within and between these two audiences, there is a resource available on my website (www.caralenapeterson.com) entitled "Questions for Starting an Internal and/or Group Dialogue about Effortless Perfection," which provides a series of prompts breaking down each of the book's six main sections so that guided conversation can happen anywhere, from the classroom to the dinner table to the dorm room.

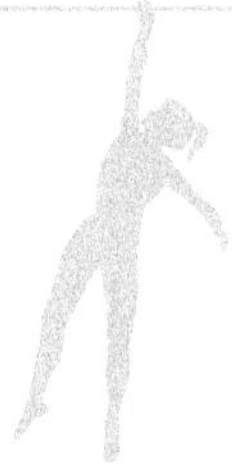

Introduction

FROM THE OUTSIDE LOOKING IN, young women are taking the country by storm. Achieving and excelling at unprecedented rates, our generation has more opportunities than any generation of women before it. We can be anything we want to be, setting our sights on jobs as lawyers, doctors, engineers, even president. Less than a hundred years ago, the number of women enrolled in institutions of higher learning that would have given them the necessary training for these positions—let alone the number of women who actually held these positions—was miniscule.

Not so true anymore.

Females now outpace males in college enrollment (a trend consistent across all races). From 1994 to 2012 alone, the share of female high school graduates enrolling in college increased 8 percent, reaching a whopping 71 percent. The share of male high school graduates enrolling in college during that same eighteen-year period stood still, remaining at 61 percent.[1]

Women also have much more to look forward to after college. The notion of attending college to land their MRS degree is becoming a distant memory. Women are in school to make lives for themselves, not to find someone willing to let them fit into theirs. Being a girl in this day and age does not mean the same thing it used to mean. The expectations are growing.

And why wouldn't they be when we appear to be delivering so thoroughly? Women have proven we *do* belong in top schools and we are *just* as fit for the working world as men are. We are becoming an increasingly unstoppable force. It is exciting and a cause for celebration! It shows that social change is possible, that cultural norms can be successfully challenged.

But—and yes, there is a but—this is the story from a distance, from the outside looking in. From the inside looking out, the story has a different feel to it. Young women are struggling in new and profound ways to keep up with the conflicting messages being sent to them by old and, now, new schools of thought. We are expected to remain feminine and communitarian (old), while competing in masculine workspaces that require advocating for oneself in a more individualized, self-focused manner to move up the success ladder (new). We are expected to meet traditional standards of beauty by staying skinny and petite like Kate Moss (old), while also developing Kardashian-style curves (new). We are expected to be chaste (old), but also sexually liberated (new). And we are expected to fall in love in a sweep-you-off-your-feet, happily-ever-after kind of way (old), while also holding tight to our career goals and never letting a partner dictate our life plans (new).

It would be one thing if the expectations placed on us were obvious, if we had a clear path to follow. Instead, we are being pinched between two paradigms that often make it impossible to succeed in compliance with one school of thought without failing in another. But that hasn't stopped us from attempting to achieve the closest possible imitation of whatever it is both these standards call for in an Effortlessly Perfect manner.

The outcomes have been devastating. Dangerous things are happening to our young, powerful, successful…vulnerable, often anxiety-ridden collegiate women. Right under our noses. Right when things have started looking up. We need to pay closer attention.

So far, I've lamented that there is a problem, but I haven't done much to address exactly what that problem is or how to fix it. My slight reluctance comes perhaps from an awareness of the kind of reactions that tend to arise when discussing issues related to gender as "gender issues." There's defensiveness, there's talk of "oversensitivity," and there's a general dismissal of gender as a serious topic.

Historically, gender issues haven't received the attention they deserve, and the practice extends to the present day. The burdens that societal expectations and biases place upon women remain largely swept under the rug, relegated to the footnotes rather than woven into the main text where they belong. Thus the struggles we face tend to be somewhat hidden from plain sight, occurring in the moments not seen by those who aren't paying full attention or don't know what to look for.

The initial statistics I presented on educational parity are encouraging, but to evaluate the state of today's collegiate women only by the numbers would be misleading. If those same researchers and statisticians were to approach each of us one by one and ask us about our private lives—our feelings of self-worth, our body images, our emotional states, and our senses of identity—a different story from the outwardly visible, surface-level statistics would become apparent: an untold story with an unspoken problem.

This is not the first time a problem of this nature has arisen. Betty Friedan launched the second wave of the feminist movement by bringing what she dubbed "the problem that has no name" into the public eye in 1963. She coined the term—and titled her book—*The Feminine Mystique,* to label the myth claiming women of that era were fulfilled by their domestic roles as wives and mothers, without any other outlets for personal expression. In reality, Friedan found many women were having mixed feelings about the lot they had been given in life, often struggling to subdue a deep disappointment with the limited traditional roles and responsibilities that they were promised would bring them fulfillment.

As women read Friedan's work, they realized that the discontent they had each individually tried to keep hidden was not something from which they alone suffered. Friedan gave women everywhere the language and the sense of solidarity they needed to discuss the impact that this unaddressed issue had on their lives and to begin planning a new future.

Looking at our present scenario, this second wave of feminism has obviously made a major difference in the expansion of women's roles and opportunities since 1963. But—there's that "but" again—an analogous form of the Feminine Mystique is still at play in a major way in the lives of today's young women. Just as was the case the first time around, this version 2.0 is not obvious to the untrained eye; hence, new language and awareness needs to be developed to address it.

In particular, we need to be more closely examining the female undergrad experience, because colleges are some of the biggest battlegrounds for those struggling against version 2.0 of the "problem that has no name"—otherwise referred to in this book as the Effortless Perfection Myth.

This book is split into multiple sections. The first, "Debunking the Effortless Perfection Myth," explains how the Myth is perpetuated while providing the basic language required to understand the concepts discussed in the rest of the book. The second section, "Perception of Self," delves into self-esteem and confidence and lays critical groundwork for the next three sections: "Reclaiming What's Ours" about assertiveness, "Taking Up Space" about body image and embodiment, and "Putting Ourselves Out There" about hookup culture and relationships. I wrap up the book with a section called "Settling into Our Identities," which delves into belonging and mental health.

Together these sections form a detailed roadmap for the empowerment of female undergrads by pointing out various manifestations of the Effortless Perfection Myth in their daily lives and considering how we as a community can approach and challenge the injustices they pose.

Let's get to work!

Section I

Debunking the Effortless Perfection Myth

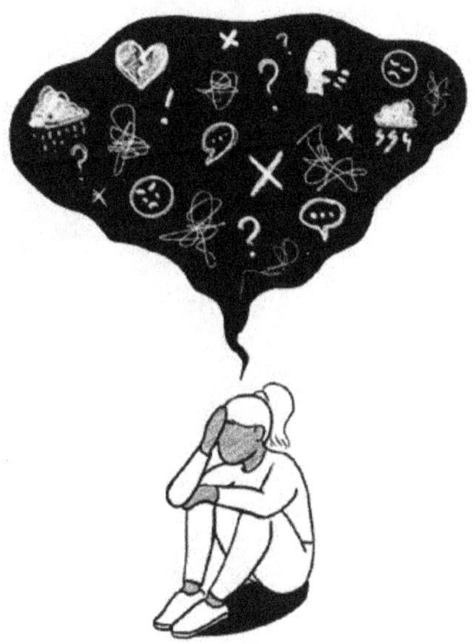

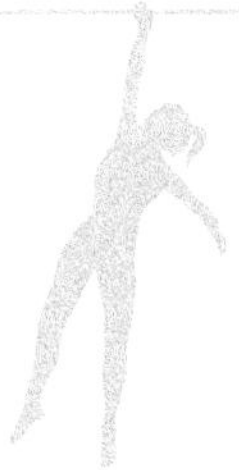

Chapter 1

The Origin Story

THE TERM "EFFORTLESS PERFECTION" has increasingly entered discourse regarding the cultural climate on college campuses over the past decade, especially in reference to undergraduate women. The term was coined in the 2003 Duke Women's Initiative Report executed under former university president Nannerl Keohane.

The report fleshes out a campus environment characterized by "the expectation that one would be smart, accomplished, fit, beautiful, and popular, and that all this would happen without visible effort." It further determines:

> *This environment enforces fairly stringent norms on undergraduate women, who feel pressure to wear fashionable (and often impractical) clothes and shoes, to diet and exercise excessively, and to hide their intelligence in order to succeed with their male peers. Being "cute" trumps being smart for women in the social environment. Men too noted pressure to wear certain kinds of clothes and adapt their bodies to certain ideals, but they felt more freedom to resist these pressures without consequences. Women who do flout the norms often remove themselves from the social mainstream, whether voluntarily or not.*
>
> *. . . The peer culture also encourages certain types of unsupportive peer relationships. Relationships with other women can revolve*

> *around women's relationship with men and can be highly competitive. Relationships with men are often sexually intimate but otherwise superficial. There is not sufficient opportunity for close relationships with peers or adults in an environment that would encourage them to resist conformity, and help create experiences affirming women's autonomy and self-determination.*[1]

The outcome of these convoluted and often polarizing dynamics is confusion among female undergrads over how to best own our power and establish ourselves socially and academically. This greatly impedes our ability to take ourselves seriously as complex individuals, which is particularly harmful during this period of our lives when we are trying to figure out what our values and goals are, what our strengths and weaknesses are, and who we want to be.

The undergrad years are anything but easy for a large percentage of today's women, yet Effortless Perfection cajoles us into hiding our complicated inner worlds by slapping on smiles and presenting personas of grace and ease to all those watching. In speaking with interviewees from a range of colleges all across the United States, I heard this point again and again. "There is an intense pressure to get good grades, be a good person, a good student, good daughter, good friend, be beautiful, and have it seem like that's all just flowing out of you as who you are and not something you constantly have to think about and live up to," explained Virginia Tech undergrad Jane.

Most claimed the pressure to appear Effortlessly Perfect had started in high school, where they felt capable of handling and even living up to its expectations; however, when they reached college, it had become too much. Vanderbilt undergrad Jordan recalls:

> *High school was when I first started experiencing it, but I didn't know at the time. I was just going about my life and didn't realize*

> *there was this "thing" driving me to be the center of social life, be involved in school, get good grades, be a "known" person—I thought that was just who I was. I never questioned it or why I felt so compelled to try so hard in all areas or how the pressure negatively impacted me.*

Then Jordan arrived at Vanderbilt and it hit her "like a freight train" that suddenly all the people around her were "just like [her] or more so—prettier, smarter, more outgoing." The thing she had been using to stand out was now the thing everyone was using to fit in. This "game" of Effortless Perfection had become one she could no longer win.

Jordan elaborates: "In college, this medal I felt like I [had] walked around with on my neck [for the past few years] wasn't special anymore and, actually, I no longer even had one." Even so, she still felt the need to compete, while simultaneously also feeling "like it was hopeless and didn't matter anymore."

She describes being compelled to do everything in overdrive until she crashed because, in trying so hard to define herself as a flawlessly, Effortlessly Perfect girl, she "lost touch with the things that really did define [her,] like being a good friend and being genuine." She wasn't alone in those feelings. Many of my interviewees exhibited similar behavior patterns—striving for Effortless Perfection at a million miles an hour until self-imploding and seriously having to reevaluate their motives.

Charlotte at High Point University painfully recalls that there was "this person [she] was trying so hard to be," and when that started to "crack," she was terrified the structure she had worked so hard to build up for basically her whole life was splintering apart. To her, Effortless Perfection was all about proving that the rules did not apply to her—that she could go out every night and party hard, but still show up to class the next day and do well on every test and assignment, while somehow having time to make it to the gym. She wanted to prove she could do everything in excess and nothing in moderation.

As her ill-fated approach to college ran its course, she remembers thinking, "I can't do this. This person is gonna fall apart and I can't be on this earth anymore. What am I if I'm not this Effortlessly Perfect version of myself that lives up to the expectations put on me by everyone else?" Charlotte's experience demonstrates how the pressures of the Myth can carry us to harsh extremes.

Jordan's and Charlotte's more personal illustrations of Effortless Perfection, along with the contextual analysis provided by the Women's Initiative Report, are helpful in getting a taste of what living within this Myth on today's college campuses is like. But nothing sums up the oppressive feeling of living in a culture of Effortless Perfection quite like the anonymous article that appeared in Duke's student-run newspaper, the *Chronicle,* just a few days after the Women's Initiative Report was released. Although this article may be viewed as a more extreme reaction to such a culture, I'd venture to say more students on America's campuses can relate to this article than cannot.

Effortless Perfection?

By Anonymous | *The Chronicle* | October 23, 2003

She was, in many ways, a typical Duke student. She enjoyed her classes, but she was smart, not brilliant. She went out occasionally, but she was at best, cute, not beautiful. She was a member of a sorority, but not one of the top tier. She was, what you could call, a "student leader;" she attended meetings with "Larry" and "Zoila" and "Nicole" [Student Affairs administrators], and generally knew what was going on on campus. She had the onion-peels-friend structure: the widest layer of natural acquaintances from classes, freshman (sic) dorm, and organizations; an inner layer of good friends from different groups; and a small core of intimate friends.

People thought she was self-assured, articulate and together. "Oh you do so much!" they said. Just like every student on campus. No one would have ever suspected she harvested anything but happiness and a prestigious degree from her Duke experience.

She worked hard on that exterior. It was important. Because what no one suspected was the demons that controlled her life, that had ravaged her self-esteem during her four years at Duke. No one realized how she felt from the moment she rolled out of bed to the early morning hours when she hit off the light. Like a failure. "Effortless perfection," the Women's Initiative called it. Female undergraduates wanted "effortless perfection." It was the new catch phrase. She didn't even want effortless perfection. Just perfection. She'd work for it. She wasn't afraid of work. But she was fixated on the ideal, and sooner or later, it all began to come undone.

She'd never been particularly self-critical or low on self-esteem in high school. Like all Duke students, she had made the grade, led the team, won the award, gotten the scholarship. But college was hard on her. She wasn't used to being asked why she would eat two bagels in one day. Or to the competitive acquisition of a new group of friends. Everyone's gotta have a BFF. Someone to call and tell you where the party's at. But wait. We're an odd numbered group, and she doesn't have one. She wasn't used to people thinking her A-minus wasn't good enough, or that wearing sweatpants in public was something to be scorned. She wasn't used to the constant reiteration that she just wasn't good enough the way she was.

So she started to change. It started out small: the desire to fit in with a certain group, to make a certain grade, to get a certain guy, to be more like a certain person. But she wavered on the edge of self-confidence, and the seemingly minute failures began to stack up, layers of bricks in the wall that slowly was pressing all the oxygen out her lungs.

Too fat. Too ugly. Too unpopular. Too weird.

Too boring. Too unhappy. Too dumb. Too scared.

Too scared to tell anyone how out of proportion the little failures had become. The little failures, the demon "almost but not quite:" the cookie eaten at 1 a.m., the A-minus on the midterm, the lack of interest following up the date. Failure boxed her in, trapped her in a roomful of mirrors confronting her with her "almost, but not quite" life. The couple holding hands. The anorexic girl buying fro-yo. The accepted job applicant. The teacher's pet.

It was the claustrophobic sense of failure that sent her to the out-of-the-way bathrooms to try to reject as much of her meal as possible without making noise. Eating marred the quest for effortless perfection. Luckily no one asked her how she got the scars on her hand. Her right front tooth, pressing down on the flesh as she thrust her hand to the back of her throat, day in, day out was the only marker of her failure. Fat people are not "effortlessly perfect." She couldn't let the cookie stay in her stomach.

Sense of failure isolated her from her friends. She felt nervy, anxious. She was a senior without career plans, the only non-banker amongst them. She watched them fly to New York and compare interview notes, and she knew she'd never make it in the corporate world. Another failure. Poor people are not effortlessly perfect. She had loans to pay. "So what are you doing next year?" they smiled and asked. "Well?" Nothing. Because she wasn't good enough.

Her lack of interest was a failure. She'd never been anything if not energetic. But now she felt different. Flaccid. Tired. People called it "senioritis." "Oh yes," she laughed, "I'm ready to graduate." But all she wanted to do was go to her room, lock out the world, lie in bed, sleep and not wake up. She didn't want anyone to see her, walking around in the baggy clothes she wore to hide the roll of stomach fat and the swinging thighs she couldn't forget. The grades she couldn't forget, the classes skipped she couldn't forget, the date functions with her girlfriends she couldn't forget. Entering the world meant walking outside to see "effortless perfection" striding across the grass, stepping on the bus, strutting down the runway. It meant seeing the world through the film of inferiority.

So on the outside she smiled and she ran and she led and she studied and she partied and she played the role of "effortless perfection" to the world. But alone in her room she hid and she ate and she threw up and ignored the phone and skipped her classes and all the meanwhile the cancerous lump in her stomach reached out insidious tentacles, poisoning an increasing number of hours, minutes, seconds. Until she started to worry her façade was going to crack. And she would have to commit the greatest failure yet: admitting there was a problem.

But she couldn't trust anyone.

So it became another worry. She worried about telling someone she had a problem. She worried about not telling

> someone she had a problem. And when she felt the worse, she worried that her roommate was going to have to walk in one day and see that she wasn't there anymore, that all the little failures had been swallowed up in a bowl of bloody water and a pink Wal-Mart razor.
>
> So she reached out in the only way she could: she wrote an anonymous editorial to *The Chronicle* the week they ran features on the Women's Initiative report, hoping, praying, that they would publish it. So that, no matter what, she wouldn't have failed to let somebody know what the Women's Initiative report never could: what it could be like to be an undergraduate woman on Duke's campus.
>
> *Editor's Note: The Chronicle holds a strict policy against running columns or letters to the editor submitted and/or intended to be run anonymously. However, we believe the column above is an extraordinary case, and we run it in this space so that those who may recognize this person may help her, and those who know people like her may help them as well. The issues the author raises affect nearly everyone at Duke, directly or indirectly, and we hope this column provokes thought, discussion and, perhaps most importantly, action.*[2]

This article poignantly demonstrates one of the most problematic byproducts of Effortless Perfection. At its worst, it can cause such intense pressure that some suffer even to the point of feeling suicidal, yet refuse to admit their reality to friends and family who could and would help. (If this is how you feel, you are not alone and you don't have to do this alone. Please do not stay quiet. Please reach out for help. Many colleges provide psychological services on their campuses. "To Write Love on Her Arms" and the Madison Holleran Foundation are also helpful resources for those struggling or those looking to support someone struggling.)

My hope in writing this book is to bring an end to the need for articles such as this one by providing access to a healthier form of relief—relief that comes from understanding the many layers of societal pressures, standards, and expectations that can really mess with our heads. I believe understanding and debunking the Effortless Perfection Myth is central to this relief. By analyzing the destructive forces directing us down a road that isn't good for us, we can begin to form a game plan that allows us to personally and collectively address the issues that often hide out under the radar.

I will be looking at these issues through a gendered lens, because my discovery of feminism and gender studies are what helped me to realize that my own negative feelings—which shared some parallels with Anonymous's story—were not fully my fault; I just didn't yet know how to push back against the things that were hurting me.

Chapter 2

Who's to Blame, "Them" or You?

I WOULD ARGUE THAT WE ALL EXPERIENCE the pressures deriving from the Effortless Perfection Myth, albeit at different points along the spectrum of severity. Make no mistake, Effortless Perfection is not just something that is cultivated in university settings, nor is it something that only applies to "elite" communities. Trace elements are present everywhere we look. The resulting toxicity begins amassing long before we get to college—in high school, middle school, even back in elementary school—when we are often programmed to turn *what we do,* and how well we do it, into *who we are.*

We transform these traits—our intellect, our athleticism, our looks, our social skills—into our full identity and obsessively chase after the approval they garner. We come to crave that approval as lifeblood because, without it, we no longer know who we are.

Except it's not that we actually have no way of knowing who we are. Rather, without external approval, we lose our gauge of who others think we are and where we stand with them. In combination with our need to earn validation from outside sources, this becomes one and the same with who we are. This mix-up causes us to jump through hoops, constantly contending with pressing internal questions such as: *What will others think of me? Will I make so-and-so proud? How can I prove my worth?* Paradoxically, these seemingly personal questions have much less to do with *us* and much more to do with *"Them."*

In this context, "Them" refers to the invisible, all-encompassing force that plays a major role in directing our lives. Women, especially, spend far too much time dedicated to pleasing this mysterious "Them." We dress ourselves in certain ways for "Them," dangerously exercise and diet for "Them," project a front of purity and innocence (while also feeling pressure to present ourselves as sexually available) for "Them," pretend the GPAs we work tirelessly to reach require next to no effort for "Them." Regardless of how well we play the complex and contradictory roles we believe are expected of us by such a demanding entity, it never seems to be enough.

Not until my last year of college, after having dutifully adhered to the Effortless Perfection Myth for several years, did it dawn on me that I was allowed to question who "Them" was and why "They" were so important. If I was going to completely exhaust myself mentally, physically, and emotionally, I should probably know why, beyond just some vague ideas: *Because this is how you've always done it. This is how things have always worked.*

So I thought about it, and I struggled with it, and I eventually came to the conclusion that all this time I had been fighting to gain validation from an empty "Them." I had allowed myself to believe that this mad pursuit of Effortless Perfection was meant to gain the approval of my parents, teachers, coaches, community, and peers (past and present). But the thing was that, for the most part, I was already in possession of all that. My parents loved me unconditionally and had outright told me on numerous occasions how proud they were of me, encouraging me to do the things that brought *me* fulfillment, as opposed to what I thought would please them. I had the respect of my teachers and coaches. I was well-liked among my peers.

All of this was also true for the majority of individuals I knew in college who struggled against the Effortless Perfection Myth alongside me. We already had a dozen sources of pride in our lives, as well as a pretty consistent flow of approval, yet one would have thought we were starved for such things, judging by the conviction with which we chased after more. We were confusing the source of our struggles.

At the heart of it all, the drive for Effortless Perfection has much less to do with gaining approval from this antagonistic "Them" and much more to do with keeping our own personal insecurities at bay. *"Them" is merely a projection of our own internal struggles, profound or not, on the rest of the world.* We have a hard time wrapping our heads around this because we don't want to believe this kind of intense pressure could be coming from within ourselves. (I acknowledge that some of us have overbearing parental figures and community standards that do impose such expectations in ways that are very distressing and unfair. But this empty "Them" theory is one I saw manifested in all my peers, at least to some extent.)

Author and spiritual leader Marianne Williamson writes, "Until we have met the monsters in ourselves, we keep trying to slay them in the outer world." Indeed, we need to learn to live with our demons, the pieces of us that bring fear and worry and regret, instead of compartmentalizing them within walls made of compliments and awards and leadership titles. In failing to do so, we are only hurting ourselves.

At the same time, I hardly believe the fault is ours. It's not as if Effortless Perfection is something to which we intentionally hand our lives over, fully willing. Given the choice, I doubt we would consciously decide to impose such a cycle of dissatisfaction upon ourselves. But, bright as we are, the Myth is so convincing that we fall prey to it. Perhaps this is because the Myth derives from a universal lie—a false promise we have long held to be true, even modeled our lives after—*that reaching perfection will ensure us security and happiness.* Thus we come to associate our flaws and imperfections with a breach in the safety and stability of our lives.

This correlation is incredibly important to understand because the concept of Effortless Perfection can often get dismissed as a petty, superficial issue based on upholding flawless appearances, when it is *so* much more than that. For many, Effortless Perfection is nothing short of survival instinct—a necessary form of self-protection, which explains why we are compelled to chase after the Myth with such fervor. The pursuit is addictive because it distracts us from the things within us that scare us most. Instead of facing our internal doubts, we adopt the Effortless Perfection Myth as our core belief system because it falsely promises to banish pain, fear, and insecurity from our lives altogether.

We embrace it, even support it among our peers, without recognizing that this mode of operation entails *being pushed by our fears as opposed to being pulled by our passions*. Our lives become all about what's not happening to us, rather than what is. Instead of existing as human *beings*, we become human *doings* perpetually stuck on hamster wheels.

Even when we catch on that the Effortless Perfection Myth is selling us a false promise, it can still be really hard to fully admit this to ourselves. To have the Effortless Perfection Myth exposed as the lie it is can be terrifying, especially when we have lived according to its bargain for so long.

But, like any addiction, to continue investing in this empty promise only ensures an even worse outcome. Because when something undesirable inevitably does happen, the Effortless Perfection Myth is set up to make us believe that it's our fault because we weren't perfect enough. So not only are we hurt by circumstance, but we convince ourselves we are entirely the ones to blame. We convince ourselves there is something wrong with us, as opposed to understanding that we are smart enough, strong enough, loved enough to deal with the ups and downs of life and that the true problem lies in the falsehoods and pressures propagated by the Myth.

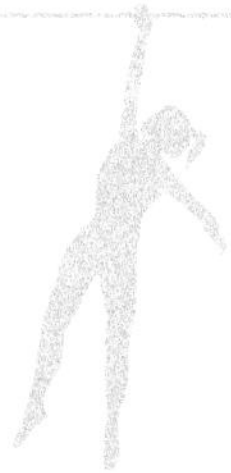

Chapter 3

Revealing the Dominant Narrative

NOW THAT WE ARE EQUIPPED with a better understanding of what the Effortless Perfection Myth is and the basics of where it derives its power, we can begin to consider our options for facing it head-on. I believe our strongest defense is learning how to identify the Myth in our everyday lives, to be cognizant of the moments in which it is impacting our perceptions, and to design a game plan for pushing back.

This isn't always as easy as it seems.

In his 2014 TEDxDuke talk, my peer Kari Barclay provides a script for a certain conversation heard over and over again on our campuses, whether riding the bus or walking to class:

> A: “How are you?”‘
> B: “I'm good. Just stressed. I have a midterm on Thursday.”
> A: “Oh, you have a midterm? I have two midterms this week.”
> B: “Two midterms? I have three papers.”
> A: “Three papers? I have four job interviews.”

Sound familiar? The exchange is humorous, but it also embodies one of the many ways students struggle with Effortless Perfection. We are so engrossed by trying to prove we are the busiest, most productive, most ahead of the game, we don't have the time or willpower to open up to others when things get a little rough. We are too preoccupied with posturing.

In fact, in 2016, researchers from Columbia, Georgetown, and Harvard found that "signaling how busy you are makes other people think you have high status" because it implicitly suggests "I am very important, and my human capital is highly sought after, which is why I'm so busy."[1]

The issue with this script is that it defines the dominant narrative on college campuses, which creates an all-too-narrow characterization:

1. Undergrads are always busy doing impressive things and being "successful."
2. Undergrads are always completely in control of their lives and everything going on within them.

So what happens when we aren't okay or things don't go as planned? After all, a lot can happen in four years. Why are we so afraid of sharing our failures and learning from them? Why are we so intent on hiding our scraped knees and wounded pride? I'd argue it's because the dominant narrative is far too convincing. Nobody is willing to reveal the pressures they feel to appear Effortlessly Perfect, so a more honest conversation never has the chance to occur.

We are all experiencing this universal pressure in one way or another, yet the large majority of us opt to carry that pressure privately without the palliative commiseration (and perhaps community-wide pushback) that honest conversation would engender. What if, instead of endlessly one-upping each other, we considered taking a step away from competition and a step toward compassion? What if, we chose to offer support, like "Ugh, I'm sorry to hear that. How are you managing all of that?"

The time has come to have a more honest and authentic conversation, to talk strategy about getting off the hamster wheel. The keystone of that strategy is understanding the dominant narrative of Effortless

Perfection on college campuses for what it is so we can begin reclaiming our agency and empowering ourselves.

Social psychologist Melanie Joy defines dominant narratives as "the stories told by the dominant culture [that] define our reality and guide our lives like an invisible hand."[2] She explains that, although these narratives are largely fictitious, they often behave like self-fulfilling prophecies. So even though the dominant narrative on a college campus may involve a way of life that runs counter to what most would otherwise desire for themselves or support for everyone else, the typical person does not think to question what they have come to see as the "natural" order. We do not see the dominant narrative for what it is—an elaborate social construction, largely manufactured and artificial.

The dominant narrative establishes itself in all sorts of ways, particularly by word of mouth (hearsay, gossip) and various forms of media (social media, television, movies, news). The image these sources project gets taken as "the facts" about the population as a whole, even though it is typically only representative of a small portion of people.

For example, most of us work hard in college, but the top 10 percent of achievers create the truly noteworthy reputation for the academic side of things (i.e. look how many Rhodes scholars we've had, look where this person got hired, look at our famous alum). By the same token, the most outrageous 10 percent of partiers will always be the ones to create the reputation for the social life side of things (i.e. make news for scandals, make themselves most visible on social media).

In both these aspects of college life, whether it be the "work hard" or the "play hard," *the out-of-the-ordinary minority gets projected as the run-of-the-mill majority because they are the most visible and, thus, draw the most attention.* As a result, they come to determine what is considered "the norm"—the unquestionable truth, the blanket statement about the main culture of a place.

Effortless Perfection has become the standard to which we all compare ourselves. We feel we are failing or falling behind if we cannot measure up to those on the extreme end of the spectrum for what intelligence or popularity or success is believed to look like in this context.

A domino effect commences when all individuals within a community choose to present themselves in accordance with the same overly publicized mold—only highlighting the parts of themselves and their experiences that best fit that mold. They talk far more about their accolades than their failures. They only upload the pictures highlighting their best nights out when they look the happiest, prettiest, and most popular. They project that they are confident and have everything figured out when, far too often, they may not feel like that at all. It is in this way that the *perceived norm* is often a far more powerful force than the *actual norm*.

The dangerous result of mistaking the perceived norm for the actual norm is a kind of campus-wide groupthink. Functions of groupthink include:

- *Illusion of unanimity*, which develops as individuals assume what appears to be the majority view or judgment is unanimous.
- *Self-censorship*, which makes it so that even if one has doubts or a desire to deviate from the perceived group consensus, they choose not to express that for fear of alienation.
- *Belief in the inherent morality of the group*, which allows individuals to feel confident in the rightness of the "cause" because so many others are going along with it, too, causing them to skip over scrutinizing the ethical and moral consequences of their decisions.[3]

Consider these elements of groupthink applied to a college campus with a constant influx of new students each fall. Every incoming class is full of freshmen longing to make their new environment feel like home, craving a sense of belonging and acceptance. The fastest route to that kind of outcome? Engaging in that same groupthink, learning what the group "ideal" is and then heavily pursuing it in hopes of fitting in, without considering potential negative outcomes of or alternatives to conformity.

As a result, *we become so set on figuring out what the culture is and how to fit into it that we don't stop to consider whether it's something we even want for ourselves in the first place.* All of this ultimately leads to the lateral loss of independent thinking, individual creativity, and unique difference within group settings.[4]

Sound like a problem? I would say so. As you might have guessed, groupthink correlates with a low probability for arriving at a successful outcome. Think about it—a culture of Effortless Perfection is definitely not a successful outcome. It's unhealthy, toxic even. It's not an outcome the majority of us who feel expected to abide by it even want for ourselves, but groupthink tells us it's a "must" or something we are "supposed to" want, so we feel compelled to go along, no questions asked.

Chapter 4

Identifying Counter-Narratives

THE FIRST STEP to pushing back against the dominant narrative of Effortless Perfection on college campuses is by identifying counter-narratives. Every dominant narrative has at least one "counter-narrative," an argument that disputes a commonly held truth or belief regarding people, cultures, and institutions.[1] Counter-narratives can be used to give a voice to those who aren't usually given one because they don't fit what has been dubbed (often incorrectly) the norm. Inclusion of counter-narratives allows these individual's experiences and perspectives to be considered as part of an overall account.

Dr. Michael Bamberg of Clark University notes that counter-narratives "do not necessarily discredit the beliefs that have been established, but instead offer a different way of thinking about particular topics."[2] These narratives often expose holes in widely accepted stereotypes by showing that they don't convey the full truth. Once we begin to establish counter-narratives, we free ourselves and others from having only one narrative, one story, one metric by which to be measured and understood.

When Effortless Perfection stands as the dominant narrative on campus with no alternatives provided, everything gets turned into an ill-fated race to gain different forms of capital that prove our worth in accordance with the Effortless Perfection standard. The social scene gets turned into an economy of social capital (be in the "right" sorority, be friends with the "right" people, go to the "best" parties). Academic pursuits are transformed into an economy of academic capital (have the highest GPA, make Dean's List, get inducted into Phi Beta Kappa). Work opportunities become an economy of work capital (get an internship at a top company, assemble the most impressive resumé). We are enclosed in a state of being that's all about establishing worth in a way that's recognizable by this system, and then we are shocked when it doesn't really leave us feeling all that fulfilled.

Longtime Harvard head of admissions William Fitzsimmons has reflected, "It is common to encounter even the most successful students, who have won all the 'prizes,' stepping back and wondering if it was all worth it. Professionals in their thirties and forties—physicians, lawyers, academics, businesspeople and others—sometimes give the impression that they are dazed survivors of some bewildering life-long boot camp."[3]

Much of the time we aren't even aware we are being sucked into this. So what's the best way to identify a dominant narrative in everyday life? Begin by asking: Are we only being provided with one "right" way to be? Are individuals being measured by a sole ideal or form of talent, as opposed to a multitude of unique gifts and contributions?[4] If the answer to these questions is yes, there's almost always a system in place that has more to do with social control and less to do with individualized agency and empowerment.

We are always in need of more counter-narratives. Social change is only made possible by those willing to bear witness to the stories outside what has been labeled dominant culture. The oppressive reality of the Effortless Perfection Myth will stand strong until we speak truth to its power and challenge its widely accepted fictions with candid facts.

Thus, I feel it's fitting to end this section with a quick look at the #HalftheStory campaign started several years ago by Vanderbilt student Larissa May. The aim of this social media awareness campaign is to "encourage individuals to share parts of their lives that exist outside of the standard social media story—life unfiltered." Four posts are included here, but I highly encourage readers to check out more via the Instagram handle @halfthestory, because this movement exhibits exactly the kind of counter-narratives we need to bring to light to combat the Effortless Perfection Myth.

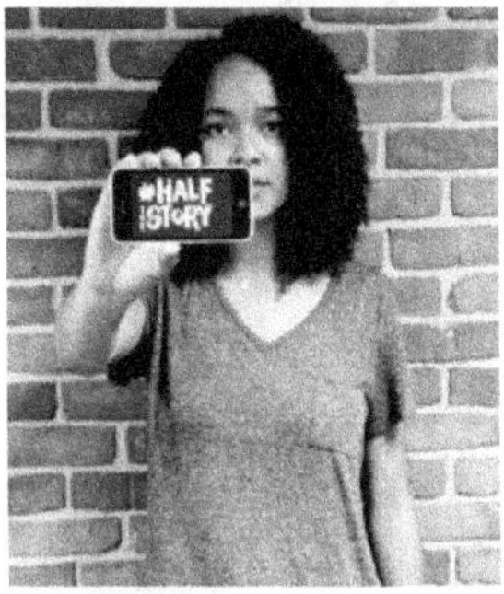

halfthestory @arianaspringflower To many people, I'm the over achiever, the over involved one, over committed, over enthusiastic...simply over- (fill in the blank). People joke and say "you're the face of Vanderbilt" and "everyone knows who you are" and I simply laugh and brush it off. I've been up front about growing up with a single mom and working hard, but this is only #halfthestory. What many of you don't know is the constant struggle behind the scenes, the anxiety I get when I see a group of people laughing and I'm alone. The fear or panic that sets in when I question if I'm doing enough or being enough or just simply if I am enough. See, I have this weird thing where I'm never satisfied, never appeased, never content. That's a great work ethic, they say. What it actually means is never-ending anxiety. So next time you see that person running themselves wild, but smiling and laughing the whole way, take a second look. You might be only seeing #halfthestory.[5]

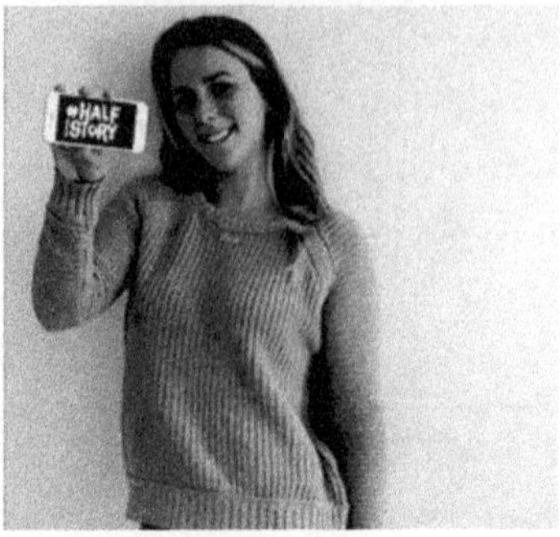

halfthestory @lucymahoney I've always been known as the athletic girl. I'm the girl who committed to play at Vanderbilt when I was a junior in high school, the girl who ran the Boston marathon, and the girl who was captain of all her sports teams. Some of you know that last year I stopped playing lacrosse at Vanderbilt, and a lot of you know it was because of my epilepsy. But what most of you don't know is what it did to me as a person. My condition eventually made it impossible to handle the stressful lifestyle of a college athlete. I started my freshmen year doing great, but then my seizures began to take over my life again and by January, my family, my neurologist and I all decided it was time to stop playing lacrosse. All of the sudden, the label that everyone, including myself, slapped on me was stripped away. I didn't know who I was without it, and all of the sudden I went from being "the great athlete" to "the epileptic." I didn't have a lot of close friends outside the team, so this was a huge adjustment and I looked into transferring to a school closer to home. Flipping through my Facebook album and my Instagram from last year, you'd think I had the best year ever, when honestly I was lost, sad, and soul searching the entire time.

I'm still soul searching today and I'm still figuring out who I am. It didn't take me long to realize that there is so much more to my identity then my commitment to sports. In the past year, I've learned more about myself then I have in most of my life. I've declared a cinema and media arts major with a double minor in studio art and corporate strategy and I plan to study abroad this summer and next fall...all things I couldn't have done being a division 1 athlete. I've learned that we shouldn't be afraid to let go of a part of ourselves that we feel we can no longer hold onto. We are meant to grow, change, and let go. I am a different person now, living a different lifestyle. And that's okay. This is my #halfthestory. What's yours?[6]

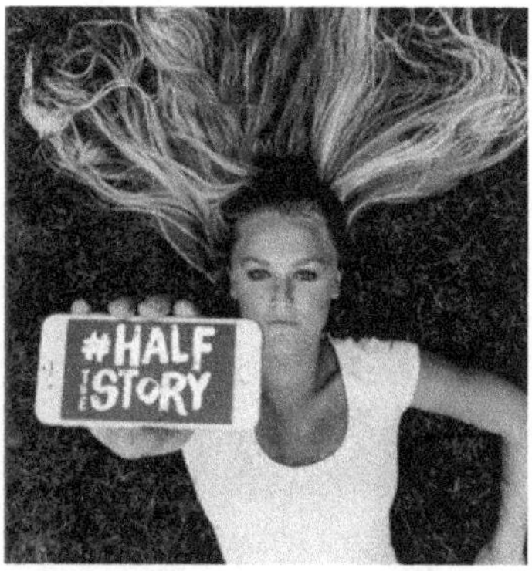

halfthestory @jacqbouchil
I go to the University of Southern California and spent my first semester abroad in Paris. During my freshmen year, my life seemed glamorous to people at home in Boston through the lens of social media. I constantly heard "Your life seems perfect!" or "You seem like you're having the time of your life!" These presumptions left me silent, and made me feel so alone. I wondered how the perception of my life, and the reality of it, were so opposite.

That freshmen year of college was the hardest of my life. Moving across the world proved to be unbelievably challenging....I realized quickly how tiny my childhood world had been, as it instantly felt so distant. The events of that year were unprecedented, as disappointment, heart break, and tragedy ceased to be even abnormal. My wisest confidant was taken by cancer. I was betrayed by the person I gave everything to. I coped with the progressing illness of a parent....I doubted who I was, and who I wanted to be, and was so overwhelmed by the sudden enormity of the unknown.

I felt myself slowly breaking that year, but none of that was on Instagram. There were montages of the beautiful places and wild adventures I had been on, but there was nothing to tell of the sadness, loneliness, or nostalgia I felt.

I realized that the essence of social media abandons the authenticity of human emotion. This distortion is closely intertwined in the mental health epidemic that faces our society today. Social media was created to unite people, but instead we are making each other feel more alone than ever. #HalftheStory is a movement that is finally promoting vulnerability and truth. Nobody should ever feel alone or ashamed in sadness, for isolation is the hardest part of personal battles against anxiety and depression. It's scary to be genuinely exposed like this, but if someone who is struggling can read this and feel less alone, isn't it worth it?[7]

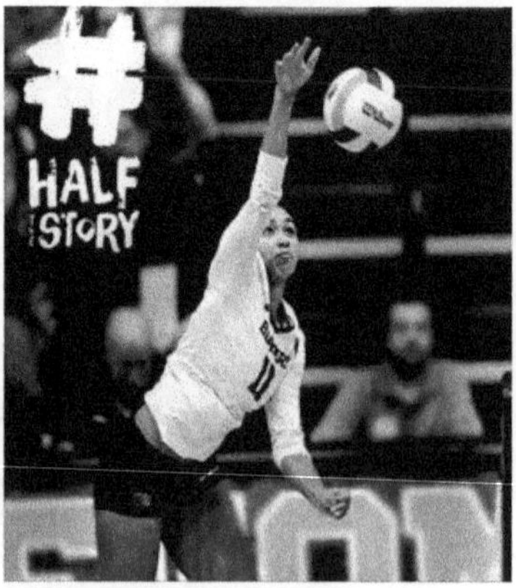

halfthestory @lanesha_reagan In high school I always felt like I had to put a mask on. I knew people expected me to act and look a certain way so I just played into that, and it was exhausting. Every day all I would do is go to school, come home for maybe an hour and then head off to club volleyball practice almost two hours away. I constantly felt isolated, and at the time it seemed like no one understood the amount of pressure I felt being a student-athlete that everyone knew of in my little town. I had amazing friends who loved me endlessly but I couldn't get on the same page as them, it felt like I was sinking further and further away from the person I was pretending to be.

It hit a moment where I was so stressed and overwhelmed by my thoughts I decided to take my own life. I took a mixture of pills and went to bed. When I woke up the next morning, I felt terrible. The pills hadn't done what I wanted in the moment and the rest of the day I felt discouraged and scared.

Later on in the day, my heart started to beat abnormally and it felt like I couldn't breathe. I asked my parents to take me to the doctor, claiming that I had chest pains. As the doctor examined me, she had to pull up my shirt to check my chest and as she did she mentioned the scar—one I made myself—that was healing on my right hip bone. While the doctor made note of the obvious self-harm mark, she said nothing else. Returning back home that day, I felt like I had hit rock bottom. Nobody was helping me when it felt like I was screaming out to them. But after that day, I woke up from the trance I was in. I finally understood that if I kept doing what I was doing, one day I wouldn't wake up.

I eventually started to find my footing. It was a hard and long process and, still, I didn't feel comfortable enough to share my struggles with others, but I did start to use healthy coping mechanisms like reading and writing.... Then, [as a student at Oregon State,] I read Madison [Holleran]'s story [a student-athlete at the University of Pennsylvania who lost her life to suicide] and it woke me up. I had to talk to someone, and I needed to keep working on being a healthier

> version of myself. I owed it to myself and everyone around me to speak up about the issues that haunted me for so long.
>
> ...I am so grateful and happy that I woke up that morning and that I got another chance to really live. I'm now a senior in college, going into my last season on the volleyball court, and I couldn't be happier that every day I get another chance to better myself. There are going to be days that feel dark, and like you are trapped underwater, but you aren't. You have to keep pushing through and, I promise, it might take time, but it will get better. #halfthestory[8]

A common thread among many of these #halfthestory posts is how the pressure to appear Effortlessly Perfect has a way of imposing an urgent drive to go, go, go. There is never a moment for pause. In the resulting frenzy, we often become so overwhelmed with the push to make ground, to lay down tracks and chug along as fast as we can, that there's no time for second thought. There's no time to sit alone with ourselves and ponder: *Why does it matter how fast I'm making ground if I never took the time to consciously choose a direction for myself?*

For example, @arianaspringflower wonders aloud in her post why it matters that she come across as the face of her school when she never feels satisfied or good enough, regardless. Sure, she is involved, she is achieving at an accelerated rate, but she's not certain if all the effort she is putting in is really delivering something that feeds her soul. Same with @lanesha_reagan, who reflects that demanding herself to be the strong student-athlete who suffers in silence is not healthy. She pushed herself forward relentlessly to fulfill the expectations she felt her small town had for her, but simply making ground didn't ensure any actual progress because she hadn't chosen a fulfilling destination.

In most of these young women's posts, the moments of pause and reflection are what allowed them to truly begin to progress because each step they made thereafter took on more intention and purpose. Whether it took removing themselves from competitive sports or enrolling in therapy, those few steps back allowed for moments of reflection and reconsideration that led to much greater strides forward later on.

Here's the thing: *If we haven't put much thought into choosing our own personal direction, it almost always means the dominant narrative has chosen that direction for us. And that direction determines more than where we end up; it determines who we become along the way.*

Of course, when the dominant narrative is Effortless Perfection, that outcome may not seem all that bad. The Myth convinces us it will provide a road map straightforward enough that we can't possibly be led astray, as long as we stick to it. But that's just a clever trap. What the Myth doesn't tell us is that to choose Effortless Perfection is to choose a default option devoid of substance. "Because all it really requires of you, mainly, is to read the zeitgeist of wherever and whenever you happen to be and assume the masks necessary to be the best at whatever the zeitgeist dictates to you," writes Anna Quindlen in her acclaimed essay "Being Perfect."[9] Sure, it feels safe to be given a template to follow. It feels even safer when that template promises you won't have to take any risks or make any choices that might bring disdain or disapproval.

But you know what it also promises you won't have to do? Think for yourself. Forge your own path. Mold your own identity. To choose Effortless Perfection is to stop following your heart because you become so set on obtaining perfection that you stop listening to the passions and pleasures beating from within your own chest.

To choose something beyond the dominant narrative of Effortless Perfection may feel like an enormous risk. But that risk is no greater than the one we would be taking by letting our lives get dictated to us by a false promise that wants nothing more than to treat us as empty vessels to be filled with its propaganda and falsehood.

Today's female undergrads generally know the right choice; we just have to consciously make it.

Deconstructing the ways in which the Effortless Perfection Myth twists and manipulates our understanding of ourselves and our environments allows us to begin unlearning the harmful beliefs and behaviors leading us down an unfulfilling path. It opens up space in our minds to actively choose what is best for ourselves instead of trusting the devious Myth to do it for us.

Now that we understand the roles of dominant and alternative narratives, and recognize that perceived norms carry a great deal of power even when they are not an accurate reflection of how a community truly feels as a whole, we can begin to address more specific issues haunting female undergrads. Of course, each of these issues still falls under the wide umbrella of the Effortless Perfection Myth.

The pressure points addressed in the remaining sections of this book include the female undergrads' relationship with self-esteem, confidence, assertiveness, body image, hookup culture, belonging, and mental health. Each plays a role in the development of our sense of identity in college and beyond.

Let's get to it!

Section II

Perception of Self

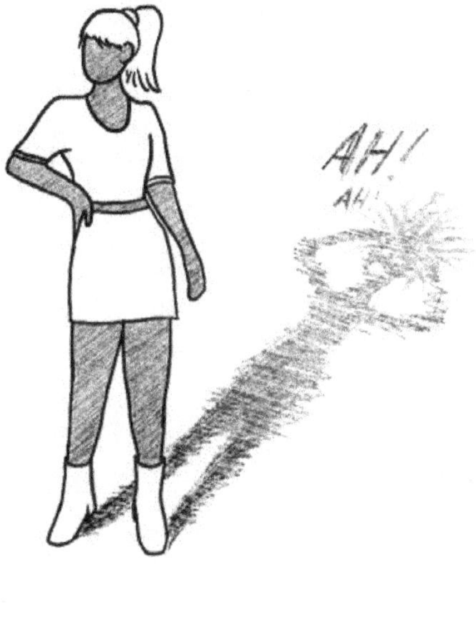

Chapter 5

Self Esteem: A Revolution from Within

ONE OF THE MOST INFLUENTIAL BOOKS I read as an undergrad was Gloria Steinem's *Revolution from Within,* a self-help text of sorts that had been published way back in 1992. I'm not sure what I was hoping to find when I pulled a copy off the shelf in a used bookstore and started reading it, but as I turned the pages it became more and more clear that the issues I was struggling with—the self-doubt, the negative body image, the fear of being anything less than Effortlessly Perfect—were not mine, alone. Steinem affirmed:

> *Wherever I traveled, I saw women who were smart, courageous, and valuable, who didn't think they were smart, courageous, or valuable—and this was true not only for women who were poor or otherwise doubly discriminated against, but for supposedly privileged and powerful women, too. It was as if the female spirit were in a garden that had grown beneath the shadows of barriers for so long that it kept growing in those same patterns, even after some of the barriers were gone.*[1]

Steinem's book made me realize that these issues had clearly been plaguing women for a long time. This epiphany simultaneously gave me relief (I was not broken! I was just like everyone else!) and made me furious (How had these things been allowed to become side effects of womanhood? We didn't deserve this!).

Steinem tied much of our plight back to self-esteem, so I began to consider that maybe I needed to start thinking about where my own sense of self-esteem came from and ways in which it might need to be restructured—which, to be honest, I never thought I'd to need to do. The concept of self-esteem had always seemed a bit hokey to me, something that preschool teachers worried about cultivating in their students by giving out an excess of gold stars. Why bother with something so elementary? I was a member of a generation of women who had been destined for success from the get-go, never having known a time before Women's Lib and able to use the opportunities the movement had afforded without a second thought. I had already proven myself over and over again in school, extracurriculars, and the social world. I didn't need a book about self-esteem! How could I—how could we—have made it as far as we had without self-esteem?!

Leave it to Steinem to show me the gaps in my thinking straight away; accomplishments do not necessarily equate to high self-esteem, especially when one is driven by an internal belief that everything one does will never be enough and there will always be more to prove (which just so happens to be Effortless Perfection's bread and butter).

Steinem drives this point home through a personal anecdote about receiving a letter from *The Keri Report: Confidence and the American Woman* informing her that, in a survey of 6,000 men and women, she had been voted one of the ten most confident women in the United States. Her reaction to this great honor? "It made me realize all over again what deep shit women were really in."[2]

Now *that* was telling.

If this champion of women's equality, this giant of social justice, didn't feel deserving of the recognition she had received (and so many felt she deserved), after all she had accomplished...well, then, I had been telling myself a lifelong lie.

I had always believed I was one step away from being truly self-assured, I just needed to accomplish XYZ and then there would be no room to question myself any longer. Once I reached those markers, I figured I'd finally feel secure as the calm, cheerful essence of Effortless Perfection washed over me. But, like Steinem, each time I accomplished XYZ, there was always a next level to pursue. The higher I got, the more I felt there was to do and the more fearful I became of losing the ground I had already won if I stopped or failed. It had never occurred to me that perhaps the reason I struggled with the concept of "being enough" had something to do with self-esteem.

It wasn't that I completely lacked self-esteem. On the contrary, I was very proud of my accomplishments and the direction in which my life seemed to be going. I had been given plenty of tools throughout my teenage years to develop a healthy, thriving sense of self-esteem. I liked who I was. But that did not stop me from experiencing the overwhelming waves of inadequacy that hit me once I got to college.

The problem wasn't so much outright esteem, but more that that esteem was contingent on so many other things outside myself—mainly the validation and approval I had grown accustomed to in high school. College was a whole new ballpark and I soon felt way out of my league: socially, academically, all of it.

Second semester of my freshman year, a junior confidant told me, "Feigned confidence is real confidence." At the time, the advice seemed spot on. I found if I just acted like I knew what I was doing, if I dressed the part and held my shoulders back a bit further, if I gave a smile and always had a drink in my hand, if I pretended to get the reference, I would come across as self-assured. I would look like I belonged, and maybe even feel like I belonged. So I worked hard at learning all the pretenses of the Effortless Perfection game.

For a period, this was enough for me. But eventually I realized that, with this feigned self-assurance, I may have been fooling others, but I certainly wasn't fooling myself. I grew exhausted from hustling for a sense of self-esteem based on approval and validation. I wanted more than this.

Because, honestly, *what was the point of it all?* What was the point of making dean's list if I still sometimes found myself doubting whether I was even smart enough to go here? What was the point of having a busy social life with tons of friends if a part of me remained forever not cool enough in my head? What was the point of starving myself stick-thin if I always felt fat? What was the point of driving myself to such extremes if the payoff was never fulfilling—was never much of a payoff at all?

I wanted to *feel* like the person everyone thought I was. If what Steinem said in her book was true, that "we create much of the outer world from within ourselves,"[3] why was I making this my reality? No matter how well I convinced people otherwise, if I felt dumb, unpopular, and fat in my head, even just part of the time, that was how I was going to experience my reality. Why was I doing this to myself?

Why were we all doing this to ourselves? I knew it wasn't just me. Once *Revolution from Within* pushed me to take off my blinders, I began to notice this bizarre Effortless Perfection–induced self-esteem epidemic all around me, manifesting itself in my female peers.

Evidence was everywhere, and painfully so. Young women too self-conscious to speak up in class, and always starting their sentences with justifiers if they did ("I'm probably wrong, but…" and "This may be a stupid question, it's just…"). Young women counting every calorie and voicing how "disgusting" they felt in their bodies through never-ending fat-talk. Young women too afraid to demand better treatment from their hookups for fear that they would end up alone at the end of the night (and oddly seeing that as the worse of the two options). Where was all this coming from? Certainly, if given a proper choice, these would not be the realities we would choose for ourselves. How much more could we be accomplishing if self-esteem weren't such an issue?

For me, the statistical "canary in the coal mine"—the warning call that goes out when something in our environment is turning toxic while managing to remain invisible—was learning that, despite all the strides that have been made, *young women continue to leave college with less self-esteem than they came in with* (while young men tend to leave with more).

One of the more recent identifications of this trend occurred at Boston College.[4] Researchers had been polling students on a variety of issues, once as freshmen and again as seniors, to track their personal development. When the trend of diminishing self-esteem for female students jumped out from the data, administrators took notice. As they delved into the data further and held discussion groups with female students, it became clear the causes were not academic (women tended to have higher GPAs). Rather, the causes were cultural, including things like body image, hookup culture, and other societal pressures.

Clearly, self-esteem is not such an elementary principle if it continues to evade so many intelligent and capable college women. So what exactly is it?

Self-esteem is "a feeling of having respect for yourself and your abilities; a confidence and satisfaction in oneself."[5] It is central to how we think of ourselves, and how we hold and present ourselves to others. At its most basic level, self-esteem is being able to agree with the statement "I am a valuable person and I feel good about myself."[6] On a grander level, self-esteem is a personal judgment of one's own overall character and the belief that he or she is worthy of love and belonging. Such beliefs are central to reaching self-actualization, yet most college women struggle to cultivate this kind of internal belief in themselves.

To be clear, I am not promoting the baseless, participation-trophy type of self-esteem. Being rewarded and praised for anything and everything, instead of genuine accomplishment and development, is a setup for grand disappointment in the future. This generation of young women doesn't need a glut of flimsy self-esteem to overcome the Effortless Perfection Myth. We need the kind of self-esteem that is rooted deep within us because we dared to travel to the center of ourselves to plant the seeds. Because we dared to do the hard work of sitting down beside the demons we harbor that inspire so much fear, and see them for what they really are—our honest needs and desires.

The truest, strongest self-esteem does not come solely from validation and approval and petty accomplishment. It arises from hard-won self-knowledge and using that self-knowledge as an empowering framework for all the ups and downs that come our way. It comes from taking the necessary steps toward becoming aware of how we are being socialized and how those natural inclinations and ways of judging ourselves, and others, are flawed.

Don't get me wrong—there are plenty of structural issues on university campuses that absolutely *must* be addressed, too. Adjustments need to be made on the institutional level. Just as one would be crazy to expect people of color to solve racism and "cure" themselves of its negative impacts without change being made on the systemic level at which it is enforced, one can't expect undergrad women to individually solve this loss of self-esteem that is no doubt impacted by the sexism experienced in their everyday lives.

The injuries we carry from the racism and sexism we experience are not our fault, but we can still involve ourselves in the rehabilitation process. Building awareness and pushing back gives us an active role to play. Knowing there are actions we can take to better our situation and the situation of others provides hope and empowerment.

Certainly, aspects of college culture pushing the Effortless Perfection Myth make it harder for our self-esteem to flourish. Shadows are still being cast where old barriers once stood. But that doesn't mean we can't venture out into those places (with our newly acquired understanding of how the Myth operates and strategies for pushing back) and try our hand at growing, perhaps even blooming.

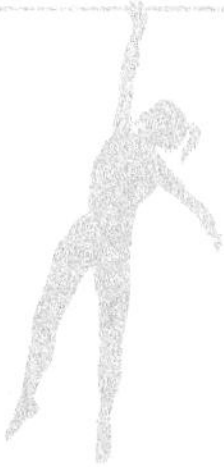

Chapter 6

Stuck Inside the "Good Girl" Trope

FOR AS LONG AS I CAN REMEMBER, I self-identified (internally, of course) as a "good girl." Probably in large part because of this, my middle and high school years were pretty much smooth sailing. I found that great things happened if I followed the straight and narrow of doing as I was told. If I fit myself into the "good girl" cookie-cutter mold prescribed by the Effortless Perfection Myth, I was ensured love, attention, and conventional success. Sure, this persona was often restricting, but the payoff felt worth it.

Once hooked, I started going to extremes to avoid all forms of conflict (which usually looked like grinning and bearing it or a great deal of over-apologizing), as the psychological cost of causing someone to feel irritated with or disappointed in me just seemed too great. If I developed any negative feelings or resentments, they had to be internalized. They did not contribute to my "good girl" image, so they weren't allowed to exist. I had to be always happy, always thankful, always smiling. Never angry, never bitter.

Many of my female peers expressed this same view. At some point, the "good girl" image became an all-encompassing identity, one that we did *not* want to lose. Abby at Northwestern explains, "I've always been a rule follower. I'm not a good liar, I don't like breaking rules, and I definitely would say fear of failure and disappointment is what drove me—especially in high school, but also college—to have a 'good girl' rep."

Mia at Georgetown mirrors this feeling: "I follow the straight and narrow and I'm terrified of authority because I don't like being in trouble." Being in trouble, after all, means being told you've made a mistake and making a mistake means you don't get to be Effortlessly Perfect.

Only two of my interviewees didn't fully identify as "good girls" (or as once having sought to fit into the "good girl" mold), though they felt that way mostly because of the role they played in their family dynamics. Both explained that, though they may have seemed like they "checked all the 'good girl' boxes," they never really defined themselves that way and neither would their parents, most likely, because they'd always been "the 'rougher' sibling, the 'wild-child' who required more attention." However, because of this, they'd felt the need to compensate in other ways, like doing really well in school or sports, or earning leadership awards and making a good impression publicly.

If they weren't able or willing to play the "good girl" role at home, they often felt double the pressure to play it outside their homes. Jordan notes, "So like, yes, I may slam my door or fight my curfew or talk back, but I will make up for it by receiving that award at school and getting into a good college and having a super-positive reputation in every other aspect of my life."

Jane felt similarly, stating that because she was the more "troublesome" child requiring more attention from her parents, she needed them to see "in other parts of my life like academics I *was* the perfect child, straight and narrow in that way."

Peggy McIntosh, former associate director of the Wellesley Centers for Women, provides psychologically based evidence as to why this drive to be "good" is such a gendered phenomenon. She notes that young girls' brains develop at an earlier age, leading them to pick up on the emotional cues encouraging them toward compliance sooner than young boys' brains tend to do. Girls start to fall in line and behave "favorably," first because we can and then because we are rewarded for it.

It doesn't take long for us to start believing we are most valuable, most lovable, when following "good girl" rules.[1]

We start craving more and more of that approval—gathering all our eggs in one basket to receive it. Because of this, *we "good girls" are missing out on experiences that are vital to building true self-esteem based on more than pleasing others*. We only become what we feel we've been granted permission to become. We don't allow ourselves the freedom of exploring alternative identities or making mistakes. When jagged edges threaten to jut out of the box we've neatly contained ourselves to, shaped by the expectations of Effortless Perfection, we clip those pieces back like hedges instead of risking to see if they bear any fruit.

Our self-esteem takes another hit as we grow older, and further gender-based socialization teaches us that it's a major gender role violation for women to be too obvious in our expressions of self-esteem.[2] "Good girl" law prohibits it. Thus, expressions associated with low self-esteem are often conflated with expressions of female altruism. Self-deprecation is sold to us as a virtue. As a result, we downplay achievements in order to get the gold star of belittlement parading as humility. We feel more comfortable underselling ourselves than boasting to a third party. We would rather be likeable as the "good girl" than risk criticism as anything else, even if that means being overlooked and underappreciated.

So, while young men are trained to present themselves as confident and self-assured regardless of the circumstances, young women are trained to be timid and self-effacing ("Who me? Oh, I'm nothing special"). And guess what—the behavior sticks. Every time we downplay our accomplishments and feign self-doubt in the presence of others, we are forming a bad habit that will stick around even when we are in the presence of nobody but ourselves. It's only a matter of time before the hardwiring of our brain sets itself to instinctively second-guess ourselves, especially when the Effortless Perfection Myth does not provide us with any alternative options, enforcing the notion that it's "good girl"-or-bust if we want to remain shiny and golden.

Lakshmi Chaudhry theorizes in her article for *The Nation* entitled "The Supergirl Syndrome" that these perfectionist pressures placed on today's women are a "transmutation of feminism."[3] She believes the revolutionary vision for women to take control of their lives and assert themselves in society was somehow absorbed into a "voraciously commercial culture intent on exploiting every aspect of human life and thought—sex, religion, race, personal identity, even feminism—to sell that new brand of toothpaste, and more importantly, to preserve the status quo."[4] Chaudhry believes the unfortunate outcome has been that women have been led to feel that respect, love, and acceptance are things that must be *earned* by transforming oneself into a sexy pin-up, valedictorian, MVP, or "preferably, all of the above."[5]

As a result, the freedom and flexibility to pursue any number of aspirations suddenly transforms into a duty to flawlessly perform and conform. Chaudhry concludes, "Women don't just need to be free to aspire; they also need to be free to just be."[6] Meanwhile, the myth being pushed by Effortless Perfection says: *You can't just be! How else will you show everyone you are worthy of their love? How else will you prove you are a "good girl" deserving of attention and respect?*

Debora Spar, former Barnard College president, iterates in her book *Wonder Women: Sex, Power, and the Quest for Perfection* that "[w]e the good girls of the 1970s, 1980s, 1990s, and 2000s" tried hard to pick up the torch feminism provided.[7] But in the process of rejecting Betty Freidan's "feminine mystique," she and her contemporaries welcomed in a new myth—the myth of "having it all."[8] She feels that doing so was a "deep and profound" failure because it just created a whole new set of unrealistic gendered expectations and constrictions. Spar advises:

> *Women of the post-feminist generation have misinterpreted feminism's call for liberation for a much more subversive quest for control. Feminism, in other words, was meant to be about expanding women's roles and choices; about giving them the freedom, for the first time in history, to participate with men as equals, and use their minds and bodies and talents, and energies as they desired. Yet somehow this expansive and revolutionary set of political goals has been squeezed—or hijacked or mistaken—into something much more narrow and personal. Rather than trying to change the world, women are obsessed too often with perfecting themselves.*[9]

Somehow, as the tides of the "feminine mystique" washed out, the tides of the Effortless Perfection Myth washed in and turned feminism into a "12-step program toward perfection."[10] Rather than banding together to form a strong collective focused on group goals like furthering opportunities for all women, many turned inward and began micromanaging themselves, picking themselves apart before giving anyone else the chance to do so.

Effortless Perfection requires us to do away with many of the unique traits and characteristics that make us who we are. After all, its mold works just the same as a cookie-cutter—churning out row after row of immaculate figurines, each one alluring but also identical. When individuality isn't present to distinguish us anymore, what's left to make us special?

We like to think that, by making ourselves as close a fit to the flawless image of the Effortlessly Perfect "good girl" as possible, we can draw in the attention we need to feel loved. It may work for a time, but eventually we will come to realize that this type of "love" comes at the terrible cost of our authenticity. Instead of choosing a genuine identity, we are choosing an imitation, and, as Anna Quindlen notes, "[N]othing important, or meaningful, or beautiful, or interesting, or great, ever came out of imitations."[11] It's just acting.

Why be loved for what you are capable of making yourself resemble when you could be loved for your uninhibited, honest self instead? There is pride to be taken in knowing you are one of a kind. The process of stepping outside the prescribed mold dictated by the Effortless Perfection Myth and being true to yourself is a noble pursuit. However, deciding to take this jump can also feel terrifying when we have been brainwashed to believe that we risk loneliness and alienation when we don't do all that we can to make ourselves "easy enough to love."

For many of my interviewees, the drive to make themselves *easy enough to love* was or had been central to their "good girl" methods of navigating the day-to-day for as long as they could remember. Edie at the University of Pennsylvania attests, "Literally my entire life—from childhood friendships to family relationships to professional partnerships—I feel like I've always tried to make other people's lives easier by silently taking things on and helping out others without admitting when I am struggling and need help, too."

She feels that this tendency toward excessive compliance has to do with wanting never to be a source of conflict and to avoid being any kind of a burden to others at all costs, even if it means making things more difficult for herself. She wishes society fostered space for women to comfortably express themselves more fully, even when the feelings they are putting out into the world are less than a happy-go-lucky, smiling, Effortlessly Perfect person. She has to coach herself through moments where she is asking for things from others, no matter how small, because being "demanding like that" makes her feel less likeable and, thus, less loveable.

For Maria at Duke, struggling to make herself "easy enough to love" circles more around her "sensitivity," which she describes as a tendency to feel her emotions, both positive and negative, more intensely than most. "I can get really excited about small things, and passionate or maybe teary-eyed. And sometimes I feel deeply about stuff that others seem to have shut themselves off to, like certain injustices or traumas, and I find myself almost feeling emotions on behalf of others," she explains.

She can't remember a time when she didn't feel like this piece of her was a barrier to being loved and earning her "good girl" status. Her impulse has always been to "dial it back" so as not to put off family members and other folks around her. She feels as though, instead of asking for the support she needs, she must tone down and hide away the sentiments she feels so viscerally if she wants to fit neatly into the box that will make it "easy" for others to love her.

Unfortunately, these efforts have had consequences for her mental health in the past. "Each time a negative reaction taught me that a part of myself was not worthy or unlovable, I would essentially cut myself off from it," she says. Eventually, she'd splintered off enough pieces that she was but a fraction of herself. As a result, her mind was constantly fighting itself because it "no longer had all the information it needed to fully function" in unison with her needs, making her even more susceptible to emotional breakdowns.

She knows that there is a middle ground. She hopes to make it there eventually, but how to go about doing so is something she is still sorting through. One thing she knows for certain is that Effortless Perfection and the "good girl" image it calls for are no friends of hers or her mental health.

For a great deal of us the Effortless Perfection Myth has infiltrated so far into our psyches that *we can't help but think of love and affection as something that we must constantly earn from others* by making ourselves smart enough, pretty enough, popular enough, agreeable enough. Instead of taking the risk of choosing for ourselves who we want to be, we let the Myth dictate our identities to us.

In the process, we are made to feel self-conscious about our quirks and outside-the-box characteristics, as though they are embarrassments to be kept behind closed doors. Are you louder than the Myth calls for? More talkative, goofy, or nerdy? Best to rein that in as much as possible. Do you have any strong convictions? You should probably keep them to yourself, lest you come off as too opinionated or strong-willed. Just play the part you were given—follow the rules dictated by the Myth, make yourself as innocuous and unobjectionable as possible. That, we learn, is the surefire way of making yourself "easy enough to love."

The ironic part is that these distinctions in character are exactly what make true affection so potent and powerful! We fall in love with the details of a person just as much as we fall in love with that person as a whole. The way their inflection changes when they invite sarcasm into the conversation, the goofy urges they act out when too highly caffeinated. The way they switch to their native tongue when schoolwork gets them stressed, causing everything to come out in a jumble of rolled Rs and harsh syllables. The way their eyes light up and their hands shoot out in wild gestures when the topic of conversation jumps to something about which they are passionate.

When I reflect on my relationships with those who mean the most to me, the most salient gifts are often the little things, the things no Myth can dictate, but that instead must rise from our natural essence. Love and affection can't fully be felt by the receiver when the receiver believes such things only come as the result of measuring up to an ideal. Or when the receiver believes every bit of love they receive must be earned through vigilant micromanagement of their own nature.

To be loved for how closely one reflects the image of Effortless Perfection is to receive a pedestal kind of love, and as Gloria Steinem so wisely attests, "a pedestal is as much a prison as any small confined space." It's isolating and lonely, regardless of how glamorous it may appear to be adored in this way. There's no sense of *I can just be me and you can just be you.* Who wants to be placed up and away from reality, when you could be held closely in the arms of those who have seen your deeper truth?

To experience real, honest-to-goodness love is to experience the freedom to be your unabashed self. It's feeling safe to let your guard down, to risk saying the wrong thing. It's being able to falter from behaving in a way you are proud of and not have that mean you are no longer worthy, because the people you call your friends are attracted to you for more than the front you put forth. They can *see* you. All of you—your good intentions, your honest efforts, your sincere vulnerability. They know you as a composite of *all* the aspects of you and are, thus, able to accept the moments in which you make mistakes. They know you well enough to give you the benefit of the doubt.

This is what waits for us on the other side of Effortless Perfection. This is why we must debunk and destroy the Myth.

Chapter 7

The Shame Game

ADDING TO THIS UPHILL BATTLE against Effortless Perfection is the way in which our desire to make ourselves "easy enough to love" makes us more prone to shame. The Myth inclines our fragile sense of self to rely strongly on external approval, so we look to others to tell us what to think of ourselves. Thus, we tend to pick up more strongly on the social cues and emotional subtleties others release during interactions. In fact, studies show women are better than men at interpreting nonverbal social cues like facial expressions, gestures, and body language to determine others' moods and emotions.[1] When something is off, we spend a great deal of time ruminating over the role we played and what we could have done differently.

This overthinking often results in "tortured cycles of useless self-recrimination" that immobilize us as we stew and beat ourselves up.[2] Susan Nolen-Hoeksema, a psychologist at Yale and author of *Women Who Think Too Much*, has found that "women have an instinct to dwell on problems rather than solutions: to spin and spin on why they did a certain thing, how well or (more often) poorly they did, and what everyone else was thinking about it."[3] *Did I come off too cocky? Should I have been more humble, more accommodating, more cheerful?* We can't stop fretting.

The perfect example is the way a number of my interviewees displayed a baffling fear of compliments. Yes, compliments! Cole, an undergrad at New York University, describes compliments as putting her in "such a vulnerable position," of all things, because "all eyes are on me with how I will react to this." She feels forced into a performance wherein she must act the perfect mix of beholden and bashful. She doesn't want to be seen as annoying by responding, "Pshaw, no I'm not," and she doesn't want to be the person always deflecting a compliment by returning, "No, *you* look good!" Focusing on how others might be perceiving her negates her ability to find her own center and to consider how she actually feels about the pleasantry she has been paid.

What does it say that many women are so distracted by what others are thinking of us that we can't even take a compliment without worrying our reaction will be misconstrued? Such preoccupations do not come from nowhere. They come from a lifetime of feeling silently judged from afar by a culture that harshly critiques us for stepping outside traditional gender roles and cultural expectations. They are an obvious side effect of shame, an emotion that is incredibly effective at making us question ourselves and our worth. Numerous psychological studies by psychologists like Dr. Tamara Ferguson and Dr. Susan Crowley at Utah State University have even pointed to evidence that "women's cultural role, greater sociability, and lower aggression, coupled with second-class citizenship, increases their tendency to experience shame."[4]

Five-time *New York Times* bestselling author and expert on vulnerability Dr. Brené Brown defines shame as "the intensely painful feeling or experience of believing that we are flawed and therefore unworthy of love and belonging."[5] She clarifies that, while shame is often seen as something reserved for those who have committed terrible acts or survived scarring traumas, it is actually something we all experience and that lurks in familiar places. Shame is a fundamental part of being human because it is so closely tied with the basic human needs of love and belonging.[6] To an extent, it's a critical emotion for informing our relationships and maintaining empathy.

Still, when shame is left unchecked, it wreaks havoc. Brown explains that the psychological impact of shame works much "like a zoom lens on a camera," so when we feel it, it is as if "the camera is zoomed in tight and all we see is our flawed selves, alone and struggling."[7] We worry we are the only ones not completely satisfied with our bodies, the only ones with complicated family lives, the only ones without serious love interests—and this experience of shame causes us to feel even further disconnected and desperate for worthiness. This sense of isolation sends us each to our own corners to privately lick the I'm-not-good-enough wounds the Effortless Perfection Myth has imposed upon us.

Charlotte reflects, "For most of college, I didn't know why I hated myself so much and then I was talking with a therapist and she was like 'you know your entire life is ruled by shame, right?'" Charlotte hadn't previously had the wherewithal to identify shame as the voice of self-doubt and unworthiness in the back of her mind, but labeling the source and realizing there was a major internal component that she could learn to control put a great deal of power back into her own hands.

When considering how shame operates in her life now, she reflects, "I think shame is a default emotion of mine. It still pops up sometimes even now after I've done all this work on myself, like when I'm on my period or not feeling good in my body or just generally operating below my typical, positive 'frequency.' I fall back into old habits and become a lot more critical of myself." When she finds that she's been knocked into a "lower vibration," she has to wake herself back up and say, "Wait a minute, I've already healed this expression. I don't tie myself to this record player anymore that's just playing the same song over and over and over again."

She considers shame an oddly "selfish" emotion in that it causes us to become very "self-focused" as we identify a negative piece of ourselves and magnify it until we lose sight of everything else. One of her tricks to overcoming this kind of "shame vortex" is concentrating on zooming back out, away from herself to more of a collective, bird's-eye view of society. That less "self-indulgent" perspective reminds her that she is far from alone in being imperfect; others are facing similar challenges and even greater ones.

The power that shame holds over us lessens when we realize that our flaws don't make us *outsiders*, they make us *insiders*. In fact, they are actually a large part of the reason why we *do* fit in, because vulnerability and shame and imperfection are fundamental parts of the human experience. Until we realize and accept this, we will misguidedly chase after Effortless Perfection as the key to belonging and worthiness.

When we seek Effortless Perfection, it is because we ache to be worthy of any number of things: popularity, respect, admiration, a seat at the table. But above all else, I think these other things are just indirect measurements we use to determine how worthy we are of that one thing we crave most—love.

The Effortless Perfection Myth takes advantage of this craving for love by promising us that, if we do exactly as it says, it will make us worthy of all the love there is to receive. It inserts itself into our weak spots and begins preaching a mentality of perfectionism that "implies a combination of rote and bloodlessness that is essentially made for machines, not men and women."[8] We become convinced that love is something we must earn from the universe, and that there's always a price to be paid in order to receive it.

Thus, we start viewing ourselves as something to be fixed, as goods that hold no value until deemed in perfect working condition—as if life operated like simple mechanics, and our hearts and our brainwaves were meant to operate as steadily as the second hand of a watch.

But we are not clocks, nor are we any form of motorized, perfunctory machinery. Love is not a matter of balancing equations; it cannot be manufactured. It is a flurry of all kinds of organic feelings and emotions that come from getting to know the actual person within, flaws and all.

How ironic that we vigorously chase after Effortless Perfection, convinced it will make us worthy of love, when it's actually our biggest enemy in achieving this goal. The Effortless Perfection Myth says: *If you can fit yourself to this flawless image, nothing can hurt you. This image will be your armor.* And the Myth speaks so loudly it drowns out the softer mutterings of true love and affection: *I can't fully give myself to you if you won't let me in. You have to trust me with the insecurities you keep secret, with the things that make you human. You have to let your walls down even if it means opening yourself to the possibility of disappointment and hurt. You have to make yourself vulnerable.*

Receiving love requires showing what's beneath the gilded front we present to the rest of the world, which, not coincidentally, is the number one thing the Effortless Perfection forbids us from doing.

In place of the notion that love must be earned, that vulnerabilities must be scorned and hidden deep, we must come to think of love as something that flows to us on our best days *and* our worst days, even when our vulnerabilities are out in the open for all to see—maybe even especially then.

After years of interviews with thousands of people on the topics of shame and worthiness, Brené Brown has found that "those who feel loveable, who love, and who experience belonging [the strongest, do so] simply because they [*believe* they] are worthy of love and belonging."[9] This belief does not come from having had better or easier lives with fewer struggles and traumas, she notes. Rather, it comes from having developed practices that help them to effectively deal with shame and hold onto their belief that they are worthy.

Some practices that I have personally found helpful include knowing my triggers for shame, speaking to myself kindly when I am feeling shame (never saying something to myself I wouldn't say to a friend), and talking through my feelings of shame with a confidant. That last practice is key because shame thrives when it is kept a secret, much the same as how the Effortless Perfection Myth thrives when nobody shares their struggles in search of palliative commiseration. As counterintuitive as it may sound, vulnerability and worthiness cannot exist without one another. Both serve as key defenses against Effortless Perfection.

Chapter 8

The Weight of "Enough"

I'LL BE THE FIRST TO ADMIT that it is not easy to navigate one's way through the shame game as a young female college student in an environment tainted by the Effortless Perfection Myth. It's as though a "good girl" isn't supposed to know her full worth, at least not outright. No wonder the word "Enough" carries so much power in the internal lives of women, especially adolescent women. I've had countless conversations about this word over the years with my female peers. Regardless of the extent of our achievements, strength of our character, or power of our presence, this word is always one we have troubled over, though the way in which we trouble over it often varies due to the source of our insecurities.

For Julie at Duke, the word "Enough" feels like an evaluation of how much she is involved with at a given time, suggesting she could always be doing more. "I often feel spread thin because I'm trying to do everything, but end up feeling like I'm not doing 'Enough' of anything," she says.

Jordan is on the same page with this assessment. Regardless of the level of success she has reached, she always finds herself worrying if it is "intense enough or prestigious enough" in the eyes of others. She notes, "My journey with the word 'Enough' is about me having to swallow the feeling of there always being some other bar I need to meet. I still struggle with just saying to myself, 'There's *no* bar, stop looking for one.'" She admits it's an urge she constantly has to keep in check.

Additionally, Jordan feels there is a piece of "Enough" that has to do with appearing to be a very specific kind of "put together" within the context of her university: "It's about being able to show up to class looking perfect and having the right answer, but also, on top of that, you need to be funny and make the teacher laugh and make that boy notice you and all the other things that go into building the persona of being the 'whole package.'"

These new expectations around "Enough" intimidated Jordan when she entered college; up to then she had been "the one who got by on appearing put together, but in a way that's like 'haha I'm quirky because I'm put together but in a messy way.'" All of a sudden the people surrounding her were "actually put together, like *really* put together." It made her self-conscious and suddenly she was internally labeling herself as too dramatic, too emotional, and too loud in a community of "true perfectionists" who somehow always managed to come off as calm, cool, and collected.

Jessie at UC–San Diego also voices resentment over being considered "too much" and having that make her feel not "Enough." Particularly as an Indian American, she explains that "there is an unspoken expectation for Indian women to just be quiet and be sort of...obedient, and I'm anything but." While she feels grateful for the richness her ethnic roots and cultural traditions have brought into her life and the lessons they have taught her, she wishes there had been a way to reap those benefits without also feeling like those around her considered her "too fierce and too passionate."

She notices that insecurities commonly arise when individuals possess traits that get them labeled as "excessive" in one way or another. It is tiring to feel that you can never entirely let loose and express yourself in the ways that feel most natural.

Jess's personal insecurities only grew in complexity as she made friends outside her Indian American community, first in her hometown of Seattle and then in college at UC–San Diego:

> *The battle of trying to be "Enough" was difficult for me because, not only was I "too much" in my loudness and outspokenness...my ethnic identity was always an issue. In my Indian community, they looked at me as "too white" (though I hate using that phrase) and with my friends, the majority of whom are white because of where I grew up and went to school, for them I was "too brown."*

Jessie attributes the strong self-esteem she has today to this constant push and pull of being "too ____" for her surroundings because it forced her to forge her own identity and her own definition of what "Enough" means to her.

In collecting all these different experiences and emotional ties regarding such a powerful word, I was particularly struck by how my interviewees discussed the concept of "Enough" either in terms of being "too much" or "too little," sometimes even both at the same time. What did it say about the pressures they were feeling that such emotions could be felt simultaneously?

Francesca at University of Alabama had the answer: "There's societal pressure to be good, smart, skinny enough, but also pressure as women not to be too smart, too funny, too anything; so 'Enough' is just finding that spot society wants you. It's finding a way to be visible and important enough for people to consider me, without having negative connotations attached." This response highlights a critically important aspect of the word "Enough"—it's tied to maintaining the status quo and the restrictive gender norms that come along with doing so.

Thus, the Effortless Perfection Myth is not so much about becoming our best selves as it is about imitating the dominant narrative.

If it were about becoming our best selves, there would be more room for emotion, exploration, creativity, and diversity. So the next time you find yourself questioning whether you are "Enough," you should use that moment to think about whether you have defined what that word means for yourself, or if you just are trying to squeeze yourself into someone else's definition.

I think the greatest part of this struggle with being "Enough" comes from the fact that many college students tend to operate according to an all-or-nothing mindset. In this mindset propagated by the Effortless Perfection Myth, there is no spectrum, just a life according to a series of binaries: yes/no, good/bad, "Enough"/worthless. Either I am, or I am not. It doesn't matter if I was a hair away from achieving the goal I wanted. Either I have made it, or I haven't.

So much of all-or-nothing thinking comes down to a desire for control and predictability—if I prove I can be it all, I will be "Enough" no matter the circumstance. We don't realize that this logic is flawed, and the opposite is actually true. Whether we feel we are "Enough" is based on the context of the circumstance, and we will never be able to predict these circumstances with absolute certainty.

So where do we go from there? How on earth is one to reach the mountaintop of "Enough" in the all-or-nothing culture created by Effortless Perfection that continuously pushes the summit higher and higher?

My personal solution has been to set my eyes on a new summit, to redirect the fight in me to a better purpose because, in the words of author and mental health advocate Hannah Brencher: "I don't want to fight to be good enough. I'm sorry, I just don't. I want to fight to make a difference. I want to fight to make it count. I want to fight to find you if you need to get found. But I don't want to fight to be enough." In other words, there are quests far more deserving of our efforts—quests about something bigger than ourselves that don't require comparison to an impossible standard or destructive competition with our peers.

Such quests acknowledge that each of us are all on different journeys. I cannot compare the leg I am on to the leg someone else is on when neither of us know what each other's journey is about.

Such quests also recognize the difference between power and strength. Power comes from an external comparison that says, "I am bigger/better/more powerful than you," while strength comes from an internal source that says, "I am big/powerful regardless." If we can focus on our inner strength, "Enough" will no longer fluctuate uncontrollably depending on relative context because "Enough" will no longer depend on the reassurance and approval of others. It will come from a stable source within.

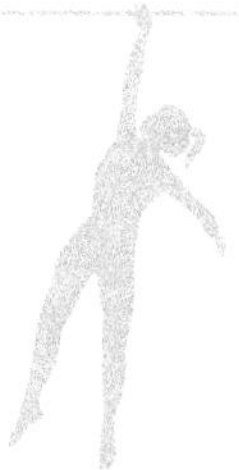

Chapter 9

Combating the Confidence Collapse

CONFIDENCE AND SELF-ESTEEM may seem like similar concepts, but they are actually two different entities. Self-esteem is tied to feelings about our worthiness, while confidence is tied to feelings about what we can achieve.[1] Thus, it is important to consider both individually.

Contrary to popular belief, confidence is about more than competition and what we outwardly project. It's not just something we make up in our heads. In actuality, it's about resoluteness of action—doing, deciding, improving. It's a sense of freedom to take risks, to aim high and assume that we have a shot at succeeding. It comes from the process of working hard, seeing it pay off, and using that to build the belief that we have what it takes to continue succeeding, which in turn propels us to take further future action in riskier and more difficult situations with higher payoffs. Ideally, this helps us build a steady foundation that also enables greater resilience following failure. The ability to bounce back instead of getting caught up in past mistakes is the ultimate prize of healthy confidence.[2]

Without confidence, we refrain from taking action. We are left on the "starting block of [our] potential."[3] Instead of focusing on trying to accomplish our dreams and desires, we spend our time and energy thinking of the dozens of reasons why we won't be able to pull them off.

Effortless Perfection is often at the root of this stalling out. The belief that we mustn't fall short of being anything-but-perfect heightens our fear of failure, which then paralyzes us into inaction. We dare not take a few bold steps into the unknown and risk a failure that may enable others to see beyond the mirage of Effortless Perfection we have carefully crafted to hide the imperfections and vulnerabilities that lie beneath.

By swearing off risk this way, we resolve never to take chances. But, as explained, taking chances is at the heart of developing a healthy confidence! The only way to overcome this fear of failure is through experiencing failure, bit by bit, until our mindset shifts and we think, "Okay, this isn't so bad; I can handle this." We must learn to take things as they come, even if we aren't sure we can handle each challenge absolutely perfectly. It's not as if that potential we are storing up is something we are accumulating interest on—it's just going to waste.

Taking risks will help us to stop holding onto Effortless Perfection as though it were a proper form of protection. Yes, it's building walls around us, and, yes, those walls may sometimes function to keep out things that could harm us. But more often those walls function to bar us from the people, places, and situations that make life fulfilling. *Effortless Perfection is not so much a protector as an overprotector*, keeping us dependent and feeding the flames of a spiraling need for external approval.

The environments cultivated on college campuses can have a way of suffocating students under a culture of Effortless Perfection. The confidence one would assume these students possess (based on past accomplishments, future projections, and so forth) is often rendered inoperative. For instance, upon returning from fall break my sophomore year, one of my closest friends revealed to me a surprising secret about the way that our college's culture made her feel about herself: "When I go home I am fine. I feel pretty and athletic and smart, just like I did in high school. But as soon as I step back on campus, I feel fat, dumb, and unpopular."

She was not alone in this feeling of deflation. In a student-run study from the 2012–2013 school year, a large portion of undergraduate women at Duke reported feeling this way:

> *When asked whether they felt more, less, or equally confident at Duke than in their home community, 41 percent of female undergrads responded that they feel less confident at Duke. In comparison, 17 percent of males feel less confident. Additionally, significantly more males than females agreed that they feel as attractive, intelligent and social as the ideal Duke student.* [4]

This report on gender and the Greek experience at Duke, called the "Greek Culture Initiative," notes that these findings are consistent with national research trends at other universities as well.[5]

For instance, Colgate undergrad Laura paints a picture of high school as having been a place of great affirmation. "What I got out of it was just a big positive feedback loop," she details. College, however, gave her more reason to question herself: "I saw my friends doing better than me in school, getting more attention from frat guys and getting invited to places I wasn't invited. I *felt* that, felt I was hanging out with lots of people I enjoyed but that didn't really *know me* yet." She struggled as she found many more reasons to question herself in college. She had to rebuild her confidence without the constant loop of affirmation she had grown so used to.

Jane similarly notes, "I felt confident walking in the door to college, but then got knocked down lots of pegs very quickly and realized I wasn't confident in really anything I was doing." She elaborates that, if she accomplished something she had worked hard for, then she felt momentarily confident, but that feeling was generally fleeting. When she would return to school after holiday breaks, she was overcome with the sense that she was "a weak person who couldn't keep up" because she missed the comfort of home so much. This anxiety "destroyed" her self-confidence for her first couple of years of college until she figured out how to overcome the cycle.

For many female undergrads, lack of confidence on campus isn't just about feeling more comfortable at home—an understandable reaction for students entering into completely new terrain. Unfortunately, their lack of confidence often remains even after they've learned the ropes in their new environments because of the problematic campus culture of Effortless Perfection they continue to encounter indefinitely.

Figures 1 and 2 are pulled from the previously discussed "Greek Culture Initiative" report. They show how members of the student population, from the freshmen to the seniors, responded to the statement "Duke's culture makes me feel confident," this time without comparison to their home communities. The findings become even more disappointing.

Figure 1
"Duke's culture makes me feel confident."

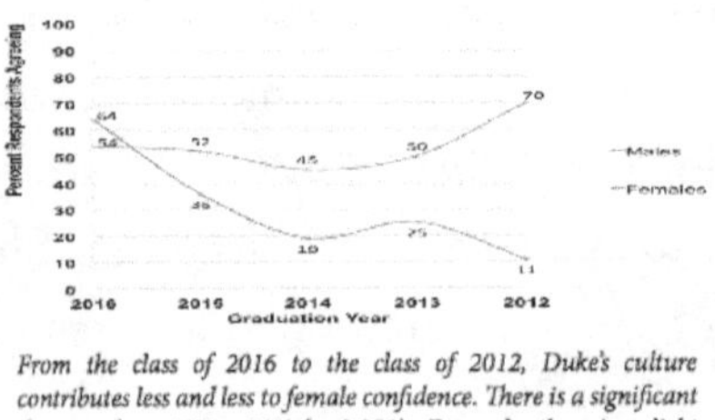

From the class of 2016 to the class of 2012, Duke's culture contributes less and less to female confidence. There is a significant decrease from 64% to 11% (p=0.000). For males there is a slight but insignificant increase in culture confidence from 54% to 70% based upon graduation year (p=0.111).

Figure 2
"Duke's culture makes me feel confident."

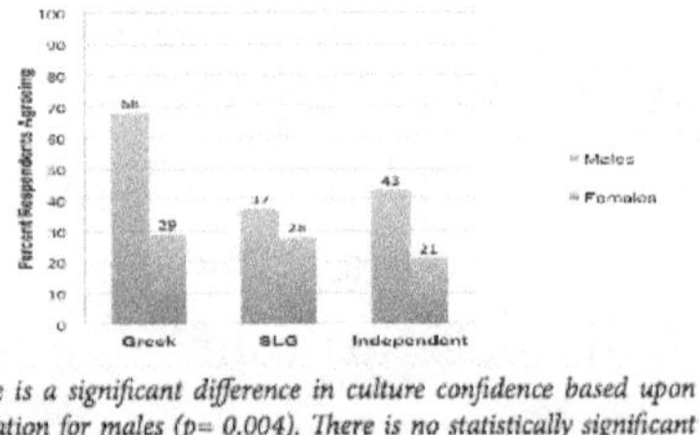

There is a significant difference in culture confidence based upon affiliation for males (p= 0.004). There is no statistically significant difference between affiliations for females (p= 0.368). The gender difference is statistically significant for Greek (p=0.000) and independent (p=0.002) students, but not for SLG students (p=0.587).

As seen in Figure 1, a dismal 11 percent of female seniors reported agreeing with the statement "Duke culture makes me feel confident," a statistically significant *decrease* of 53 percentage points from the 64 percent of female freshmen who agreed with this statement. On the other hand, 70 percent of male seniors agreed with the statement, a statistically insignificant *increase* from the 54 percent of male freshmen.[6] To frame this another way, at the end of their college experience, close to seven in 10 of the males surveyed claimed the school's culture made them feel confident and only one in ten females did.

Figure 2 breaks down this same information by gender and social affiliation with all four years of students (freshmen through seniors) combined. The study claims there is no statistically significant difference in confidence according to social affiliation (Greek Life, Selective Living Group, or Independent) for women. The data does show, however, that across the board, regardless of affiliation, men appear to feel more confidence than women—particularly Greek men—within their various affiliations. No matter how one spins the data, the average female ends up with lower confidence than her average male counterpart at the end of four years (not to mention *during* the majority of those years).

These statistics are not exclusive to Duke. The 2012 Boston College study noted in Chapter 5 on self-esteem showed the same results, and there are more studies just like it. The Harvard Project on the Psychology of Women and Development of Girls had similar findings back in the 1970s, as did the work of Dr. Patricia Coughlin at Northwestern, who reflects, "My research, published in 1984, in the *Journal of Personality and Social Psychology*, revealed an anti-developmental trend in females throughout their college years. They entered college in a secure and confident state and tended to leave in an insecure and anxious state. How sad to see this continues decades later."[7] Sad indeed.

How do we push back against the confidence collapse caused by the Effortless Perfection Myth? We begin by inspecting why our confidence is so vulnerable to collapse in the first place.[i] After my own thorough examination, and the guidance of my college psychologist Gary Glass, I've learned shaky up-and-down confidence is typically linked to "reassurance addictions," or the constant need to self-validate (a problem that stems from self-perception issues discussed in Chapters 6 and 7).

Such reassurance addictions function by causing us to stop trusting our own judgment when it comes to personal worth, which is why grades and other quantitative forms of measurement become such a fixation. We believe that if we can get a mark—on paper!—that verifies our achievements, then the doubts buzzing around our minds will be quieted, at least momentarily. Only the appraisals with accompanying proof seem to matter, as a gnawing suspicion that nothing else is to be trusted grows inside us.

In this way, our achievement-oriented mindsets tend to put us at risk for chasing after accomplishment as if it were a cure-all. We say to ourselves, *I will be "Enough" once I __________ (get this GPA, lose this weight, am dating this person, am a part of this social group). Only then will I be truly happy.* But this mindset always pushes contentedness into the future and makes it dependent on utopian circumstances. We find ourselves incessantly chasing after a hollow trophy.

The Effortless Perfection Myth reinforces our reassurance addictions by encouraging us to go after more, more, more as a way of ensuring we are doing everything possible to achieve the best, most flawlessly beautiful trajectory for our lives. We are pushed by the fear that if we don't take advantage of every last opportunity, we will find ourselves on a path that is "lesser." We must "do it all" so that we are never cut off

[i] In addition to these individual efforts, we all should collectively be demanding a more supportive environment for female students from our institutions of higher learning. Such demands might include hiring more female faculty, creating or allocating more funds to a women's center on campus, prioritizing speakers who address gender-specific issues as part of their platform, and reconsidering housing assignments that prioritize fraternity housing to the most desired parts of campus (to name a few). The more trustees, administrators, and alum we can get on board, the better!

from possibilities that may ensure us a happier, more recognizably successful life in the future. We reason that the ability to make *any* choice means we should eventually be able to make the *best* choice when the time comes.[8] But nobody knows when that moment will actually arrive and what it will look like.

We aren't thinking about contentedness as something created in the moment. We are guided by the idea that by compiling "more"—more titles, more awards, more followers on Instagram—we will have eventually compiled enough social, academic, and economic capital that we can exchange it for joy and purpose. But that's just not how life works.

After all, confidence that comes from the rank our achievements afford us, and other external forms of recognition, is almost always precarious. It remains based on conformity to someone else's standards, just like with self-esteem. There needs to be passion and intention behind our actions.

For instance, Jane was doing "extremely well" in college, pursuing two degrees and on track to graduate with honors. However, she still felt these external achievements did nothing to cure her anxious and hopeless feelings. She notes, "Even when I knew in my heart that it wasn't working, I still kept going on this notion that I had to do this, I had to achieve because my achievement would eventually, one day, fix everything." Despite knowing her approach was misguided, she was too afraid to stop for fear that things would get worse before they got better.

Jordan similarly reflects, "When you feel there are gaps in you or things that aren't how you want them to be, the easiest way to feel like you are making ground and fixing that can be to accomplish something." At the same time, she believes that if the root of the problem isn't that you are a "lazy sloth of a person" (and odds are if your solution to problems is to accomplish something, you are likely not a lazy sloth of a person) than that achievement is just acting as a Band-Aid.

In both scenarios, we find that confidence and accomplishment do not always go hand in hand. We have to be going after those accomplishments for the right reasons. Accomplishment is not a cure-all. I repeat, *accomplishment is not a cure-all.*

In an article called "Don't Send Your Kid to the Ivy League," William Deresiewicz warns, "[T]he nation's top colleges are turning our kids into zombies."[9] His statements tie clearly to the Effortless Perfection Myth, particularly his statements about the trip lines surrounding confidence and accomplishment within highly competitive university environments:

> *Our system of elite education manufactures young people who are smart and talented and driven, yes, but also anxious, timid, and lost, with little intellectual curiosity and a stunted sense of purpose: trapped in a bubble of privilege, heading meekly in the same direction, great at what they're doing but with no idea why they're doing it. Look beneath the façade of seamless well-adjustment, and what you often find are toxic levels of fear, anxiety, and depression, of emptiness and aimlessness and isolation....*
>
> *So extreme are the admission standards now that kids who manage to get into elite colleges have, by definition, never experienced anything but success. The prospect of not being successful terrifies them, disorients them. The cost of falling short, even temporarily, becomes not merely practical, but existential. The result is a violent aversion to risk. You have no margin for error, so you avoid the possibility that you will ever make an error.*[10]

Deresiewicz's statements support what I've been driving home this whole time, that the culture of our high-pressure university environments is stifling the very foundation of confidence building, through the enforcement of the Effortless Perfection Myth. College women, especially, don't feel they can take the risks necessary to develop a resilient confidence because failure has become so taboo. Instead, our confidence remains brittle and easily broken.

Chapter 10

Fear of Failure: More Debilitating than Failure Itself

UPON FIRST GLANCE, those in lockstep with the Effortless Perfect Myth are hyper-successful, self-assured individuals ready to take on the world—what one might call "Confidence Incarnate." However, closer inspection reveals Effortless Perfection to be Confidence Incarnate's evil twin. They may look identical, but one has a dark side.

Beyond its dangerous pull toward reassurance addiction, the dark side of Effortless Perfection paints failure as something to be avoided at all costs. In contrast, the truly confident among us—those whose belief in themselves and their abilities doesn't come and go like the tide—recognize failure as an ally, not an enemy. They do not see it as the end of the road, in the way that a devotee of Effortless Perfection does, but rather as a necessary part of reaching their fullest potential and building a resilient confidence.

Of all the questions I asked my interviewees, the one that brought the most deeply reflective, heartfelt responses was: *When was the first time you felt like you truly failed? Did it come as late as college?* For most of them, failure—true failure that cut deep—was not something they had experienced until they were freshmen, sophomores, or even juniors in undergrad. And when it had happened, it wasn't typically just a spur-of-the-moment thing. It was the result of stress and pressure and fear and anxiety that had been building up for years.

Jane claims her first true "failure" occurred her junior year, the day she was supposed to drive back to Virginia Tech after a holiday break: "My parents were out and all I needed to do was get in my car and go. I backed out of the driveway, went twenty feet and suddenly was like, I *cannot* move. I can't press the gas pedal." She sat in her car for several hours unable to free herself from the anxiety that left her frozen.

Eventually, Jane was able to cajole herself to park the car back on her driveway, go inside, and call her parents. "I felt so much shame calling them and just being like, 'I'm *done* and I need to figure something out,'" she says. "I mean, they knew I struggled with anxiety, but they didn't realize how bad it had gotten....In that moment, I felt like I'd failed everything I'd been working towards. It was all over, *I was done.* What was I going to do with my life? Like, what happened to me? My whole identity was gone."

With time, Jane realized that she just needed to face the issue head-on by asking for help, and that this was nothing of which to be ashamed. She still graduated on time, and with honors. It wasn't by any means the end of her life, even though the intense buildup of never having really failed before made it feel that way in the moment.

Her misstep had been assuming that confidence came from outrunning failure, from never having to look failure in the eye. In reality, it was her lack of experience with failure that made her confidence so brittle. Finding herself face to face with it in this way gave her no other option than to let it break her down, but then being broken down gave her the opportunity to witness her own ability to build herself back up. She hadn't expected that. She was much stronger than she'd realized.

Her life had momentarily veered out of control, but she'd handled it. And watching herself handle it—observing this messier, grittier, far-from-perfect inner identity make itself known—was deeply empowering. Moving forward, she knew that ferocity was within her. She recognized that she need not fear failure because that part of herself would always be there. With this knowledge, her confidence evolved from a shaky, fragile thing to a resilient, dependable force with which to be reckoned.

Charlotte had a somewhat similar story to Jane. Her big crisis moment also presented itself as a panic attack her junior year while on a holiday break. Though, her sense of failure did not come so much from the panic attack itself, as her inability to stop it without drugs:

> *I was lying on the floor in my house... at school I had been heavily using all kinds of things to get rid of this feeling when it came, but at home I didn't have anything to use. My dad walked in and had never seen me like that. My parents took me out of school for two weeks. It was a whole conversation of whether I could mentally handle going back. And the sense of failure was just coming from all sides: I'd failed at hiding all this shit that was really inside me, failed academically being pulled out of school, failed with how out of control my drug use had gotten.*

She'd hit her rock bottom. "I felt totally helpless, like, fuck, I'm actually a broken human. The vase dropped and shattered and it was up to me to find a way to glue it all back together, and to do it right this time," she says.

Like Jane, Charlotte also made it through this struggle. She returned to school after spending time in a rehabilitation center. She reflects that her senior year "after figuring so much out" was by far her favorite, most meaningful year of college. By finally allowing herself a moment to pause, get help, and reevaluate, she found she was suddenly free to take her life in a different, healthier direction.

Furthermore, she felt more confident in her ability to survive hardship. Before, she hadn't met the fiercely intuitive, spiritually resourceful side of herself that emerged when it came time to heal and push through her scary anxious feelings without the assistance of a substance. Meeting that part of herself imbued her with the kind of resilient confidence that did not cower in the face of addiction. Anxiety and depression were no longer signs of imminent failure, but hardships she was fully capable of living with and moving through.

While not all of my interviewees struggled with Effortless Perfection to the point that it extended this deeply into their mental health, the majority felt greatly impacted by it nonetheless. I can't stress enough that the pressure caused by Effortless Perfection is not just some silly little nuisance. It is a true mental health concern. I myself can attest to its ability to drag us into an entirely different state of mind where obsession with achievement and image are blown out of proportion, and fear of failure pushes us to extremes we never thought we'd reach.

My first big experience with failure took place my sophomore year of college when I pushed my brain too hard studying for a statistics final and it shut down thirty minutes into the big test. The stress I'd been putting on myself caused me to max out and I essentially lost my ability to read for a three-hour window.

After hobbling through the questions as best I could, I turned in my test packet and beelined straight to my dorm room, where I closed the door, sank to the floor, and immediately broke down into heavy sobs. This wasn't some *I can't do this, it's too hard* breakdown. It was an *I'm scared, what is happening to me?!* breakdown. I had never failed a test before, let alone a final. I had never thought that it was possible to push myself too hard, or that I actually had a breaking point. "This is just about mental toughness," I'd always said to myself, and kept going. Until now, that had always worked.

But this was different. Over the next three days, I started having full-blown anxiety attacks whenever I tried to get some sleep. My mind was too scared to let me doze off because it knew there was work I could be doing. I feared that my exam fiasco was a bad omen for *every mental challenge I would take on for the rest of my life.* That's right—I thought that if I had failed this one time, nothing would stop me from failing over and over again *for the rest of my life.* I was convinced my time as the smart-studious-college-student-full-of-potential was crashing to a halt, like I'd lost the right to make it a part of my identity anymore. Talk about the opposite of a resilient confidence!

Thankfully, I worked up the courage to take my first trip to CAPS (Counseling and Psychological Services). I walked myself to the office, went up to the front desk, and said: "I don't have an appointment, but I really need to see someone. I think I'm having a nervous breakdown." As I was explaining the situation to the psychologist, I started hyperventilating, so he handed me a paper bag to breathe into and advised me, in the understatement of the year, "You need to seriously think about the kind of pressure you put on yourself."

I know now he was trying to take some of the stress off my back by suggesting I deserved to give myself a break every now and then. But, in the moment, I felt like he was saying that this meltdown clearly showed I couldn't hold myself together and perform academically the way everyone else here could. I no longer fit the mold of "the norm." I was different from the average student at my school. My shiny exterior had developed a crack and I had to learn to settle for second-rate.

Of course, the psychologist hadn't even come close to saying *any* of this. But the Effortless Perfection Myth had deeply affected my perception of the things I was seeing and hearing all around me. *Under the guise of protecting me from failure, it was in fact prompting me to see myself as a failure.* It was priming me to feel isolated and alone in my struggle.

Only later did I discover that these perceptions could not have been more false. Given adequate time to reflect, I learned several important things from this experience: *There are indeed limits. Burnout is a real thing. Balance is non-negotiable. It's okay to ask for help.*

Over time, my experiences with failure no longer had such stark repercussions on my mental health because the sensation came to feel more and more normalized. My increasing confidence in my ability to work through failure meant that my fear of it was no longer so paralyzing.

As William Deresiewicz has written, "If your standards are as high as they should be, you will fail again and again."[1] Total invincibility should not be the goal because it is simply not possible. Today's collegiate women need to find a way to trust that failure is not synonymous with being a "broken human" who is "done" and "destined to fail at every mental challenge for the rest of [her] life," as Jane, Charlotte, and I were so quick to assume. We need to open ourselves up more fully to learning the lessons of how to fail, how to *really* fail and accept it as a normal part of life, and trust that letting our imperfections show will not derail our future.

After listening to so many deeply personal accounts about struggling to build more resilient confidence, I was thrilled when I finally found an interviewee who expressed a truly healthy, long-term relationship with failure. Blake at Pitzer College said she couldn't recall any "big significant moment" when she felt she had failed because she'd met "a lot of small, more consistent failures" throughout her life. She mainly attributes her healthy confidence to her involvement in sports. "Maybe you don't make the big championship game, or you do, but the game goes into triple overtime and you miss the winning goal," she explains. Either way, "you just have to learn to shrug it off and work harder for the next time."

Blake's experiences are very much in line with the overall findings of psychological studies regarding failure and confidence development. Nansook Park, an expert in psychology at the University of Michigan, explains in *The Confidence Code*, "The proper way to build confidence in children is to offer them graduated exposure to risk."[2] If taken in one big dose, it can be disarming and traumatic. But if absorbed gradually over time, failure can be the equivalent of a series of inoculations.

Blake spoke to this issue as well. She recalled watching friends go to college and really struggle—to the point of having identity crises—with no longer being the smartest kid in the class. But, she explained, "I had never been the smartest kid in the class. I always worked hard and did well, but it wasn't about being the best, it was just about doing *my* best." Blake's healthy attitude toward failure allowed her to flourish as an undergrad because she entered with a fundamental understanding that running away from all possible forms of failure isn't an option. She developed a mindset that was able to pull herself out of the nitty-gritty and see the bigger picture. She knew how to be incredibly driven, while also knowing when to cut herself slack.

As a recovering perfectionist, I've employed numerous strategies for working toward a similarly healthy mindset and a more resilient confidence. For instance, I still like to write out goals for myself at the start of each year and revisit them every two months or so to check my progress, but I have adapted my behavior to make sure I'm not ever looking only at all the things I have *yet* to accomplish. When I reach a milestone or accomplish a task on my "to-do" list, instead of crossing it off, I move it to a separate list of things already accomplished that year. When I'm being too hard on myself or struggling with a recent failure, I can revisit this list to remind myself that I still have a great deal to be proud of.

This system allows me to hold myself accountable, while also protecting my confidence in my ability to get things done and bolstering my desire to keep trying when some goals take longer to accomplish than hoped or expected. I'm less focused on the next rung on the ladder and more focused on the big picture.

Furthermore, my to-do list incorporates "resumé goals," which are related to career hopes and dreams, as well as "eulogy goals," which are related to the kind of person I want to be and how I hope to be remembered once I am gone. By putting something like "publish article with *Ms. Magazine*" on the same list as "host a dinner party once a month to connect with various friend groups," I am reminded that both of these things hold importance in living the kind of purposeful life I want to live. I am able to push back against the "accomplishment-as-cure" mindset imposed by the Effortless Perfection Myth by prioritizing more than just the things that will supposedly mark me as "good enough" in the eyes of others.

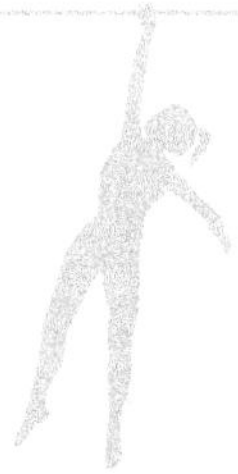

Chapter 11

C's Get Degrees

CONFIDENCE IS NOT THE KIND OF THING you either have or you don't; it's built over time. Many of today's collegiate women have a hard time accepting this and I think it's because the Effortless Perfection Myth leads us to believe we should somehow be able to achieve and succeed without the input of intense work or strain. As Psychologist Stephen Hinshaw expounds in his book *The Triple Bind*, "A girl who works hard on her looks and her sex appeal is a bitch, a slut, or simply shallow. A girl who takes her studies seriously is a bookworm, a brain, or a nerd....[And a] girl who actively pursues a boy of her choice is pathetic."[1] In these scenarios, effort is a mark of inadequacy, something to be scorned.

After years of providing mental health services and therapy to adolescent women, Dr. Hinshaw's professional experiences have led him to believe this unfortunate association between effort and social taboo occurs because women are often expected to "present their appearance, their abilities, and their unique identities, not as the product of enormous labor but as the 'natural' expression of their inner beauty."[2] Ugh.

We've got a major problem, here. *When effort is taken out of the equation, all these personal skill sets and traits are seen as qualities that either you have or you don't.* The major downfall with this way of thinking is that a girl who believes intelligence (and other adaptable, elastic traits) is a fixed, inborn quality—as Effortless Perfection would have her believe—assumes upon failing at a task that she must just be stupid (or ugly or unathletic or boring), rather than considering she might just need to increase her focus and work harder.[3] If she were to see her accomplishments as the fruits of her efforts, she would continue to feel empowered, even when stumbling over roadblocks here and there; this resulting kind of resilient confidence should be the goal. Unfortunately, we have a long way to go to get to that goal.

One place where this particularly applies is the STEM fields (science, technology, engineering, math). Two new research studies have found that female students might be abandoning STEM majors that would likely lead to more profitable professions later in life because they are terrified of getting anything lower than an A (and humanities classes do not tend to grade as harshly as STEM classes).[4] The inability to do something "perfectly" scares us away.

Harvard economics professor Claudia Goldin wanted to know why so few women major in her field; only 29 percent of bachelor's degrees in economics go to women.[5] Examining grades in her introductory economics classes, she found that the likelihood a woman would go on to major in economics often corresponded with how well she did in that one intro class. As her grade fell, the likelihood she would remain in the major fell, too. A woman who received a B in Econ 101 was half as likely to stick with the discipline as a woman who received an A. Here is the kicker: Professor Goldin's study found there was no such trend for the men. Men who received B's were just as likely to continue to pursue economics as those who received A's.

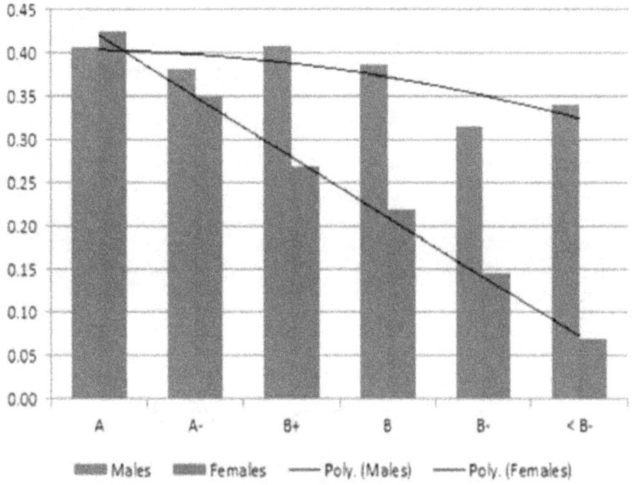

This chart shows the percentage of male and female students who received a given grade in introductory economics course who then later majored in economics. Data refer to an anonymous research institution, from a study by Harvard Professor Claudia Goldin. (Claudia Goldin/Harvard University)[6]

A similar trend has been found with women in engineering. In 2012, *U.S. News* reported that female students often drop out of engineering programs with higher average grades than male students who stay in engineering programs.[7]

Dr. Goldin is quoted in Catherine Rampell's *Washington Post* article "Women Shouldn't Chase after A's in College to Make More Later":

> *Maybe women just don't want to get things wrong.... They don't want to walk around being a B-minus student in something. They want to find something they can be an A student in. They want something where the professor will pat them on the back and say 'You're doing so well!' [Whereas g]uys don't seem to give two damns. They just have their eyes on the prize.*[8]

When the Effortless Perfection Myth is at play, women are reluctant to be anything but perfect because to be not perfect is to be not

"Enough," and to be not "Enough" means not appeasing the reassurance addictions we have incorporated into our cores. We crave a pat on the back, a top grade, a high GPA to retain our sense of certainty and security. We fear being a B– student will somehow make us a B– person.[9]

But running away from failure in this way is limiting. We are straying away from the very opportunities we need to build a more resilient confidence that has been tested. We are hurting ourselves in the long run, not to mention causing a major brain drain in the STEM fields that our society and our futures can't afford!

Dave Dunning, a professor of psychology at Cornell, builds upon Goldin's remarks when suggesting that, beyond fear of receiving less than perfect grades, women sometimes drop harder classes and majors because we have a greater tendency to personalize and internalize setbacks. Dunning has noticed, "Men in [a harder] course recognize the hurdle for what it is and respond to their lower grades by saying, 'Wow, this is a tough course.'" This kind of response is otherwise known as *external attribution*, usually a healthy sign of resilient confidence. On the other hand, Dunning observes that for women, "When the course gets hard for them, their reaction is, 'You see, I knew I wasn't good enough.'" This kind of response is known as *internal attribution*, and is usually debilitating in situations involving failure.[10]

Internal attribution was exactly my response when falling short on my statistics final. Instead of thinking, "Okay, I probably pushed myself too hard on that one," I actually questioned whether I was smart enough to attend my university. Piper, a STEM student at Pitzer, shared that same unhealthy reaction when struggling through the ultimate weed-out class for biochemistry and pre-med hopefuls—organic chemistry. She received a "low grade notice" halfway through the impossibly hard class and her immediate reaction was "I'm not smart enough. I just can't read fast enough. I can't comprehend well enough. Why did I think I could do this?"

The heart of this problem is that men and women are socialized to attribute their successes and failures to different things. Numerous studies show that when a boy succeeds he most often sees it as due to skill (therefore, taking steps toward building confidence), whereas girls are more likely to attribute successes to luck, help received, or amount of effort put in (keeping confidence level). When a boy fails, he tends to see it as lack of effort or an unlucky situation and takes it in stride (keeping confidence level). Girls are more likely to attribute failure to a fault in themselves, a lack of skill rather than a lack of effort, or just bad luck (thus lowering confidence).[11] What this ultimately means is that, as girls, we give ourselves no room to make up ground. Good things keep us even; bad things drag us down. We only allow ourselves to stay put, at best.

We need to stop evaluating ourselves like an exam where we start with one hundred points and, each time we get a question wrong, our score goes down. Instead, we should be scoring ourselves more like a basketball game where we are constantly putting points on the board. Maybe we miss an easy layup every now and then, but we always have the opportunity to steal the ball back. There's inherent forgiveness in adopting this perspective instead of succumbing to the staggering fear that our mistakes will permanently affect the final outcome, or that a single blunder means "game over." The Effortless Perfection Myth only holds onto its power so long as we refuse to believe failures and mistakes are just part of the game.

Chapter 12

Stereotype Threat and Imposter Syndrome

PRIOR TO WRITING THIS BOOK, I commonly found myself wondering: Why do women's confidence meters seem so faulty and finicky in comparison to men's confidence meters? When assessing the environmental factors of each situation we are in—pressures, expectations, and so forth—how are the reads men and women are getting so different? For instance, how can a single blunder—like getting a bad grade in an intro to economics class—make such an impact on a female undergrad's confidence that she would rather switch majors than continue to pursue the subject? How come a male undergrad who makes a similar blunder stays the course so seemingly unaffected?

I think it's because, even when men and women occupy the same space, their experiences of that space are different based on what they feel is expected of them. The way women view and value ourselves is correlated to how the societies and groups to which we belong view and value us. Men and women continue to be valued in different ways for different things, which alters the gendered expectations placed on us. We are not expected to pursue economics or other male-dominated majors, so we have a heightened awareness of all the little signs telling us we don't belong—signs that the guys probably aren't even registering because they don't have their guard up in the same way due to fear of gendered stereotyping.

Gender stereotypes may seem like water under the bridge, or some pesky little mosquito that women either need to squash early on or learn to ignore, but it's not that simple. Stereotypes and prejudices are complicated in the way they reveal themselves. Psychological studies have shown that they really do impact how we see, feel, and behave, even when we *think* we are paying them no mind.

Psychologists use the term "stereotype threat" to label the tendency of those who fear confirming a negative stereotype, based on their social group or identity markers, to confirm it nonetheless because their fear triggers an internal bias (against themselves) that causes subpar performance.[1]

Dr. Claude Steele and Dr. Joshua Aronson coined the term in 1995 after performing several experiments showing, when race was emphasized (even just by the checking of a box), Black students performed more poorly on standardized tests than white students. They found that, when race was not emphasized, this gap in performance decreased dramatically and concluded that "performance in academic contexts can be harmed by the awareness that one's behavior might be viewed through the lens of racial stereotypes."[2]

Since this original study in 1995, the influence of stereotype threat has been explored through numerous other studies. It has been found to harm the academic performance of Hispanic students, students from low socioeconomic backgrounds, female students in math, and even white males "when faced with the specter of Asian superiority in math."[3] Beyond academics, stereotype threat has been shown to impact typical everyday behaviors like women negotiating, women driving, and white men playing sports.

As a female computer science major at the University of Maryland, Melissa describes having experienced stereotype threat: "Seventy to 80 percent of my major is male, so I felt a lot of shame on my end, freshman and sophomore year, around making mistakes in class because I felt like, well, if I get an answer wrong people might think, 'Of course she did. She's a girl, what's she doing here?'"

Melissa's anxieties no doubt impacted her ability to perform to the best of her ability. In her mind, only Effortless Perfection would suffice if she wanted to prove that she really belonged. She fretted over asking questions for fear of appearing like she couldn't keep up, and was distracted from committing her full focus to her work while stressing about how she was being perceived. Her confidence suffered as she developed a heightened fear of failure that held her back from taking risks and challenging herself.

As other women in the major with whom she had formed friendships and study groups dropped out one by one—suddenly saying they "just didn't want to do it anymore"—Melissa couldn't help but think that maybe she should drop too. "There were so many times sitting in class, I thought to myself: These people don't look or talk like me. I can't do this. This isn't for me. There's no way I'm going to succeed."(A somewhat valid concern seeing as studies have found women tend to perform less well and drop out more often than men in classes where they represent a minority, and make more progress in courses with higher proportions of women.)[4] At the same time, she felt passionate about the subject matter and attests that passion was what helped her to adopt a new frame of mind: "You just have to have this mentality of 'I belong here and I deserve this.'"

But such an approach to stereotype threat doesn't work for everyone, especially when stereotype threat has been known to take away the confidence even to attempt to prove inaccurate biases wrong. Dr. Zachary Estes, a research psychologist at the University of Warwick, demonstrated this phenomenon in a study wherein he gave roughly 550 students a series of tests in which they were instructed to reorganize 3-D images on a computer screen. The first time the students took the test, the women scored measurably worse than the men, thus confirming the gender stereotype that women are worse than men at spatial relations (which help with things like sports and driving). But upon looking at this first round of results more closely, Estes found the biggest reason women had done poorly wasn't that they were making more mistakes; rather, the women hadn't even attempted to answer a large portion of the questions in the first place!

Estes gave the test again, this time instructing participants to at least try to solve all of the problems. The end results showed women's scores increasing sharply to the point that they actually matched the men's. *Lack of confidence in correlation with stereotype threat—not lack of ability—had gotten the best of the female participants.*[5] The women's inaction, their choice (conscious or subconscious) not to try, was the culprit.

Stereotypes matter because expectations matter. When we stereotype women as less proficient in math, science, and technology, we automatically expect them to do less well. When we expect them to do less well, they are far more likely to do exactly that. In fact, studies have shown that the higher overall gender equity is in a country, the smaller the gender gaps are in math.[6] Given the right support, women do just as well as men—there isn't some inherent difference in ability depending on one's sex.

The uphill battle that women fight to maintain a healthy level of confidence is also complicated by "imposter syndrome," which entails a tendency to have counterintuitive reactions to praise for one's accomplishments. "Instead of feeling worthy of recognition, we feel undeserving and guilty, as if a mistake has been made," Sheryl Sandberg explains in *Lean In.*[7]

Francesca at the University of Alabama knows the feelings associated with imposter syndrome all too well. When applying for a Fulbright Scholarship her senior year, she was in "a constant state of questioning." She explains, "I went through this process of thinking,

'Who do I think I am that I can get this?' and feeling conceited to be applying for the scholarship." She wasn't even so much worried about her qualifications as she was worried what people would think of her for thinking she was good enough to apply for a Fulbright. "And if Fulbright did pick me," she worried, "like, would they have meant to pick me?"

Francesca did end up being awarded a Fulbright in the end, but still notes having to make an effort to break out of the harmful thinking that imposter syndrome continues to force upon her. "I read somewhere that when looking at job descriptions, a guy will apply if he meets 60 percent of the requirements, but girls feel the need to fit 100 percent before they'll consider applying," she says. (The study she's referring to is from a widely circulated 2014 Hewlett Packard internal report.)[8] She reminds herself of this all the time so as not to become a part of the statistic. She need not be 100 percent perfect just to throw her hat in the ring. Her work performance need not be 100 percent effortless to try for a scholarship or promotion.

Even as high achievers, many successful women struggle to shake the feeling they are about to be "found out" at any minute. Ironically, it is those highest on the totem pole who tend to experience this the worst. Kate Bahn notes in her article "Faking It: Women, Academia, and Impostor Syndrome," "In order to feel like you're faking it, you need to have already reached a certain level in your discipline. Think of it as a twisted version of the Socratic paradox—the more you know, the more you feel like you know nothing."[9] The more successful we become, the less successful we feel. Not so reassuring, is it?

The issue of imposter syndrome can be even more of a hurdle for women of color, notes Jessie. "Sometimes people make us feel like we are here or got the opportunities we did because someone needed to fill the diversity box, so we should just be happy for what we have and not push for more," she explains. She believes if women have to work twice as hard to be recognized and feel confident, women of color have to work three times as hard.

Imposter syndrome grows in its complexity as identity markers like race and socioeconomic status intersect with the politics of gender. In predominantly white environments, women of color are often simultaneously hyper-visible and hyper-invisible. Studies show good work or positive behavior is less likely to be acknowledged, and bad work or negative behavior draws amplified attention.[10]

For instance, studies also show "Black women are more harshly evaluated under conditions of organizational failure when compared with Black men, white men, and white women due to the 'double jeopardy' effect."[11] That "double jeopardy" exists because, in the U.S., most publicly recognized leaders belong to dominant groups when it comes to their identity markers; they are either white (dominant racial group) or male (dominant gender group). Because this is what we are most used to as a society, our concept of an effective, typical leader is closely associated with whiteness and maleness, which causes unconscious bias against those who don't fit the expected mold. Because Black women are neither male nor white, they face a double bias in this respect.

Such bias not only threatens that they will receive harsher judgment when things at their organization go wrong, but it also threatens that they will pay a stronger penalty for their mistakes.[12] This unbalanced and unfair scrutiny further feeds fear of failure because women of color know they will not always be allowed the same number of mistakes as their white or male peers. As a result, their confidence suffers in part because they aren't provided with the same opportunities to build the kind of resilient confidence that comes from being given enough leeway to test limits, fall down, and get back up again.

First-generation college students and those from low-income families also tend to have a heightened sense of imposter syndrome. A friend of mine at Duke noted experiencing imposter syndrome because those around her seemed to have completely different relationships with money. They did not seem to have to worry about it ever, while money worries were constantly occupying her mind. She felt like an outsider who was living inside the campus walls but observing the goings-on with the sense that she was somehow still peering over a gate.

Another peer said that, because she was the first member of her family to attend college, she didn't know how to take advantage of opportunities in the same way that individuals with parents who had the institutional knowledge of a college grad could. She felt like an imposter because others could ask their parents for first-hand advice, while she was just making it up as she went along. She struggled to develop a resilient confidence because she did not have the same safety net to catch her, making her timid in the face of new challenges. She had greater difficultly becoming a betting woman, even when the thing she was betting on was herself.

Stereotype threat and imposter syndrome are very real hazards for women's confidence that cause us consistently to underestimate ourselves. They are part of the reason that numerous studies spanning the past twenty-five years show female students self-estimating their intelligence as much lower than their male peers, [13] while also maintaining higher average grades.[14] What purpose does such self-doubt serve?

Is it possible that the not-good-enough mantra of the Effortless Perfection Myth has infiltrated so far into our psyches that we've started beating ourselves up before it can?

Or is it that the pipeline for female leadership is so small that only those who seem to possess superwoman strength make it through, while the rest of us look at them in awe as we struggle to identify with the

Effortless Perfection they project and we fear ourselves to be lacking?

Perhaps it is both. Maybe women routinely underestimate and sell ourselves short because we don't feel we can be given full credit for our accomplishments if we have made mistakes along the way—believing only flawlessness deserves that kind of recognition. Only Effortless Perfection truly counts for anything in our minds. Thus, we feel the need to camouflage our cracks and hairline fractures from others when, actually, these struggles may be exactly what those younger than us, looking up to us as role models and mentors, need to see.

As a female majoring in biochemistry, Piper at Pitzer College notes, "I have a hard time thinking of who my college role models have been—two or three female professors and maybe a female TA who was very nice and explained things to me. But, no, I wouldn't say I ever heard about them struggling with anything." She reflects on finding through a Google search that one of her few female professors had already been working toward her PhD at nineteen years of age. Another female professor she'd had was head of her department, taught multiple classes, mothered three kids, and even played D-I athletics back in college.

Piper comments, "I tried to see how she did it and I couldn't really figure it out. With all my female professors, I watch them and their mannerisms and how they react to pressure and stress—they are calm, cool, and collected and I'm just trying to be like that." But it is hard for Piper to feel like she can ever reach the level of success that these women have reached, likely in part because they fit the stereotype of Effortless Perfection and, in her mind, she does not.

Katie at Northwestern was able to feel differently from Piper because she had previously experienced a mentor she admired discuss her vulnerabilities openly. She'd gone on a retreat where one of the slightly older co-facilitators shared that she had dealt with disordered eating earlier in her life. Katie recalls, "When she opened up about body image, it totally hit home for me because it made me feel like it was okay for me to share, too, and it fostered this great environment for all the girls on the trip where we all started sharing and having these realizations."

Just one person in a leadership role opening up allowed all the girls to feel like they could open up, too. Her ability to be confident in spite of her flaws and insecurities gave them the permission to be confident by the same right. Overcoming hardship became a source of pride and respect, as opposed to appearing flawlessly unmarked by struggle, thus diminishing the effect of Effortless Perfection.

Similarly, Jordan's big epiphany came when one of the girls she admired in her sorority, a girl who eventually became her "Big," opened up about her private struggles. As Jordan explains, she was one of those people who "appeared to have everything—she was the prettiest girl in our sorority, she had a super-hot boyfriend, and an adorable dog and lived in this awesome apartment, and was nice and always smiling." However, as the two got closer and had more in-depth conversations about life on campus, her "Big" opened up about struggling with significant depression for which she'd been hospitalized multiple times. "It's really eye-opening." Jordan continues, "when a person you idolize as having it all suddenly reveals to you that they don't because it shows you the hollowness of this Effortlessly Perfect front so many of us are desperately trying to build for ourselves." The experience helped her see reality a bit more clearly.

In my opinion, we don't need superwomen to help move us forward into bigger and better opportunities. We need authentic, sincere women who are willing to be honest about the struggles they ran into to get to where they are so the other women following after them realize that they are allowed to struggle, too, and that struggle doesn't make any of us any less worthy.

A small piece of the Effortless Perfection Myth unravels every time we open our mouths and share what we are going through. By all means, we should be setting our goals high and striving to make an impact, but we also need to remember to *show enough of our own vulnerabilities that others do not feel the need to hide their own*. When we tell our success stories, we should also remind those listening that there will always be bumps in the road—that is normal and to be expected.

Chapter 13

Elect Her

THE STRUGGLE WOMEN FACE when trying to develop a healthy, resilient confidence becomes an even bigger issue when considering that confidence is often mistaken for competence.[1] Our society is drawn to charismatic, confident leaders because they embody a sureness in themselves that makes us feel like we can sit back and let them take the reins. Unfortunately, many talented and capable potential female leaders are riddled with self-doubt that holds them back from inspiring the same kind of trust.

We need to be able to trust *ourselves* first. If we can't convince ourselves of our own qualifications, how are we meant to convince others? To run for a high-profile leadership position on campus, like young trustee or student body president, one must be willing to self-promote and to face the possibility of failure. The Effortless Perfection Myth makes that hard.

"Women still see themselves as outsiders. They don't see themselves as already being at the table," writes Kate Farrar of the American Association of University Women.[2] As a result, we require much more encouragement and support from others even to consider running for a leadership role. Research shows we tend to wait to be asked to run as opposed to internally deriving the confidence to make that decision ourselves.[3]

Katie recalls an interview with a congresswoman she did as part of a young women's empowerment program called She Rocks the World, wherein this *national* leader confessed she hadn't been planning on running for the position until a male colleague of hers announced publicly at a large event that indeed she was. She'd been too afraid to take the risk, to move her family, until "someone pushed [her] into the pool." The congresswoman encouraged the She Rocks the World ambassadors not to be afraid of taking similar risks especially since "we are not naturally inclined to do that as girls in this society."

Julie, who served as student body president her junior year of college, expressed similar feelings. "I'm fairly risk averse, so I didn't run until I felt much more sure than not that if I ran I would win," she reflects. She canvassed all potential candidates and only decided to run once she knew certain other people wouldn't run, so it would be an easier fight for her. Julie may not have needed someone else to tell her to run, but timidness toward going after leadership positions still played a role in her decision-making. She felt the natural inclination to hold back and admits that pressures surrounding Effortless Perfection may have played a part in this.

The *Washington Post* reported in 2011, "At the 50 colleges ranked highest by *U.S. News & World Report*, less than a third of student presidents are women."[4] This statistic is important beyond the university setting because women who are engaged in politics and elected to offices earlier in life are more likely to continue along this route. Don't forget—confidence is built by taking on challenges and seeing our potential with our own eyes, and it increases as one engages in more and more challenging experiences. Politics are no exception.

Jennifer Lawless, director of the Women and Politics Institute at American University, and Richard Fox, a political science professor at Loyola Marymount University, conducted a research project that found individuals who run for student office are 11 percentage points more likely to run for political office later in life.[5] In fact, according to a report released in 2013 by the Scholars Strategy Network, 40 percent of women in Congress at the time were first involved in student government.[6]

This is definitely something to keep in mind when, in the 60–100 years women have been able to vote in our country (only white women won the right to vote in 1920), the stats for female representation remain abysmal. As of 2021, only 45 women have ever served as state governors, and 20 states still have never had a female governor.[7] Only 6 women have ever served on the Supreme Court (there have been nearly 120 justices since its founding). The year 2021 saw a record high of female representation in Congress at 27% (a 50% increase from just one decade ago).[8] And there is yet to be a female president.

When considering the statistics for women of color, things only get worse. Only 2 state governors have been women of color.[9] Only one Supreme Court Justice has ever been a woman of color. Only 6 women of color have ever served in the Senate (there are 100 senators serving at any given time); and only 83 women of color have ever served in the House (there are 435 house representatives serving at any given time).[10]

Fortunately, there are groups committed to change. The American Association of University Women, Running Start, and She Should Run started collaborating on a national initiative called Elect Her in 2009. This initiative is dedicated to building a pipeline of women running for public office by starting at the college level. Running Start has been running the project solo since 2016.

Caroline Heldman, a professor of political science at Occidental College, says in the documentary *Miss Representation* that when children are seven years old, an equal number of boys and girls—roughly 30 percent—express a desire to be president when they grow up, but when you ask them again at fifteen, a massive gap emerges. She notes with great distress that this demonstrates our country's "gendered socialization where politics is considered to be for men, leadership is considered to be a masculine pursuit, and women are discouraged from pursuing ambitious positions."[11]

Elect Her is very much aware, in the face of these gender stereotypes and biases, that female politicians (both in their younger and older years) require more encouragement to run than their male counterparts.[12] Not surprisingly, the curriculum of Elect Her workshops focuses on building confidence—the confidence to claim credit for work accomplished, the confidence to self-advocate, the confidence to run without needing to be asked, the confidence to assert oneself and take a potentially unpopular position on an issue. Women tend to find all of these competencies more difficult than men do. My hunch, as usual, is that much of this has to do with Effortless Perfection and subsequent gender role restrictions, as discussed in previous chapters.

Overall, this trend of females lacking the confidence to launch themselves into the political world hurts everyone, not just women, because those who could serve the best aren't always the ones reaching for the jobs. The world doesn't get to benefit from their talents. Women continue to be robbed of role models in higher ranks and the cycle of male-dominated leadership continues. As the saying goes, "It's not who you are that's holding you back, it's who you think you're not." The time has come to own our talents and all that we have to contribute. Someone has to get the job done—why not have it be us?

Fun fact: Elect Her made a visit to Duke in 2012 and the subsequent increase we had in female representation suggests it made a big impact. From 1996 to 2011, only two of the sixteen student government presidents were women. Then, starting in 2012, we had four in a row (three of whom were women of color). Just think, there's a class of students at Duke who will never know what it's like to have had a male student body president. This has been the case countless time in reverse, with students not knowing what it's like to have a female president. How cool is it these women have been able to flip that trend on its head?!

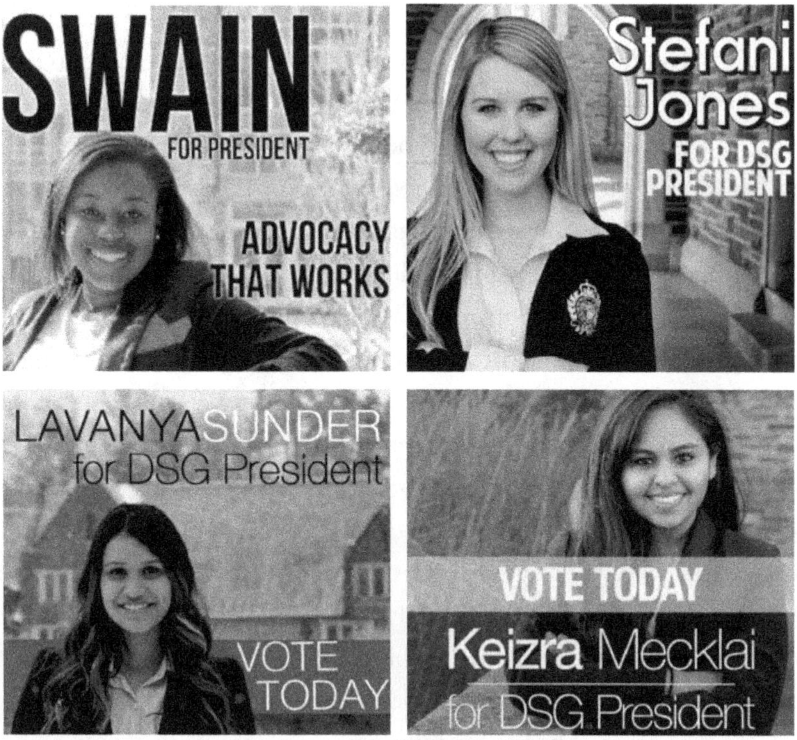

If there is a campus you think could benefit from an Elect Her workshop, reach out to them via runningstart.org. Since 2009, over 300 Elect Her trainings have been held at over 120 schools in 40 states for more than 9,500 students.

It is critical that we find a way to bring greater diversity into the spaces where political decisions are made. Having an equitable number of females in leadership positions is vital. In her TED Talk "The Credibility Gap: How Sexism Shapes Human Knowledge," Soraya Chemaly argues that, when a narrow segment of the population gets to make decisions for the entirety of that population, it is not only disappointing but is "deeply immoral."[13] She stresses that it does not matter if every individual in that group is a wonderful person with the best of intentions, aiming to make ethical decisions. There will still remain an "epistemological flaw" within the makeup of the governing body because it is "simply not diverse enough to capture what we need to capture for the world to be a more just place."[14] In short, diverse representation matters.

It matters because we naturally place more weight on the issues that impact us the most personally. When a female undergrad is elected to student body president or a similar position of influence on campus, gender issues are more likely to be addressed during her time in office. A male is less likely to feel strongly about female-specific issues, like access to birth control via student health or justice for victims of gender-based violence, because if those rights and protections were to disappear, his life arguably wouldn't change all that much. A woman's life, on the other hand, *would* change, maybe even drastically, so her concern is more likely to come with a sense of urgency behind it, thus making it more likely to impact how she votes or what campaign issues she prioritizes.

By that same token, a heterosexual cisgender person is less likely to recognize the full importance of LGBTQ-specific rights and protections on campus, such as access to gender-neutral housing and restrooms or adequate funding for an LGBTQ center.

Empathy is not the same as experience. Awareness of an issue is not the same as possessing the urgent drive to change it. We need more women, people of color, people with diverse gender identities and sexual orientations, and people of different socioeconomic statuses involved at the core of our country's decision-making processes—everywhere from college campuses to our nation's capital. Having minorities in mind is different from actually knowing what it is like to be one. We need the seats at the table to be filled with a more diverse makeup if we want our society to work best for all, instead of a select few.

If being in student government or serving as young trustee or running for elected office in the future is something that interests you as a collegiate woman, you are doing yourself and society a disservice by not giving it a try. If nothing else, we must all be confident in our unique ability to bring a diverse and necessary perspective to the table. The judgment we have felt and the lies we have allowed ourselves to believe at the hands of the Effortless Perfection Myth are holding us back. We must remind ourselves that we may not be perfect, but neither are the people we are running against! All we can do is bring to the table what we've got and give it our best shot.

Chapter 14

Feminizing What Confidence Can Look Like

THE EFFORTLESS PERFECTION MYTH places very stringent demands on how collegiate women should and should not act. Sometimes, those demands are just as *contradictory* as they are stringent. One of the most obvious testaments to the mixed messages women receive regarding the "right" and "wrong" ways to successfully empower ourselves is the double-bind around confidence. We are encouraged to act more confident, but when we finally do project that confidence, it isn't always well-received. This damned-if-you-do-damned-if-you-don't predicament arises from the way in which our society's traditional understanding of what confidence looks is, in part, gendered.

"There is a completely different idea of what a confident woman looks like versus a confident man. It's so much easier for women to step over the line between being confident 'enough' and being 'too' confident," Francesca laments.

Abby agrees: "Confidence is *one hundred percent* gendered. Let me tell ya, males are just given room to be cockier. They can use more inappropriate humor and curse words, and they are allowed a more 'swaggy' confidence than women." As a student-athlete, she is very aware of how women are judged differently than their male counterparts for outward expressions of pride and celebration of skill both on and off the court.

The general consensus from each of my interviewees was that male confidence is allowed to exist in a more "unbridled" state, whereas women must be cautious with how they let it show. This assessment particularly hit home for Edie, who felt that if there was one big lesson she learned in high school it was "toning down [her] confidence in exchange for greater likability among [her] peers and also [her] teachers."

She describes coming to high school as "an above-average-on-the-confidence-spectrum kind of girl" with a certain level of pride in herself coming out as "natural expression." Sadly, this was not well-received. She recalls running into a great deal of pushback: "Edie is conceited, they would say. Or Edie is cocky. Edie is arrogant." Looking back on this period of her life objectively, she really doesn't feel like she was doing anything out of line. "I wasn't broadcasting that I thought I was the best, or gloating when I achieved something. I just wasn't criticizing myself or cutting myself down and that wasn't the norm for most girls. It wasn't expected," she notes.

What frustrates her more than anything is knowing that the men in her class who projected similar fronts of confidence (and perhaps even more so) received the opposite response from those around them. Their projection of confidence made them "like a magnet" where everyone from fellow students to administrative figures were drawn to them. Yet her confidence was "a matter of friction." The guys were encouraged to develop a confident persona, while she learned life would be easier if she repressed that aspect of herself. (Edie's personal observations are backed by implicit-bias studies showing that when girls do not hedge their speech, when they assert their opinions without apology, adults see them as "rude," "confrontational," "uncooperative," and "transgressive.")[1]

The commentary from Francesca, Abby, and Edie reminds me of a panel of six student-athletes I was on in high school. One guy on the panel was singing his own praises about his 4.0 GPA and accomplishments on the court, and I remember thinking to myself that never in a million years would I feel okay with openly giving myself kudos in such a way for fear I'd be labeled as ridiculously conceited. It's against the rules of being an Effortlessly Perfect "good girl" to know your worth, after all! But for him, it just seemed to work.

I brought up this scenario while interviewing Jane. She just nodded and said, "Girls' confidence is supposed to be internalized. It's almost not good to be super confident because, if you are, you are stuck up. You are supposed to downplay achievements. There's this delicate balance that I feel like guys don't worry about—they are allowed to say it like it is and we can't." Expressing confidence as a woman is a complicated dance. No wonder so many of us would rather just refrain from expressing it at all.

Is it possible that some of these complications arise because confidence is defined more with a male in mind? The authors of *The Confidence Code* draw attention to this important point:

> *Male workplace bravado—perhaps testosterone-fueled and* Mad Men*-inspired—is still the gold standard. It is currently the only standard. The drive to win no matter the cost. The boundless craving for risk. The propensity for quick decisions. The emphasis on high-decibel and high-energy interaction. Those are values and methods of behaving.*[2]

Yet, when women try to act according to these values and methods of behaving, they are often assessed quite negatively. What gives?! Why doesn't this most widely recognized definition of confidence leave any space for us?

There are many things women can do on their own to combat the Effortless Perfection Myth, but this is one area where we undeniably need help. As a society, we have a collective responsibility to rework our understanding of confidence to include space for women. We need to question ourselves and others when turned off by a woman stating a strong opinion or asserting herself. We should be asking, "Would we feel turned off like this if a man were acting the same way?" and "How might our implicit biases be impacting our interpretation of this situation?"

Furthermore, we need to recognize and appreciate the ways many women have created their own alternative, nuanced manners of expressing confidence. Some of us don't feel comfortable projecting confidence in a stereotypical, traditionally male way because doing so feels like wearing a phony suit of armor. We want to stay true to what feels personally authentic—and that's totally okay.

One thing we each *can* do individually as women is to decide what honest, authentic confidence looks like for each of us, personally. Maybe it looks like bringing attention to the good work of our team on a project, referring to the success in terms of "we" more than "I," but at least including ourselves. Maybe it looks like supporting female peers by negotiating assertively for each other. (Research has actually shown that women perform better when advocating for others as opposed to when advocating for themselves, whereas men's behavior doesn't tend to shift depending on who they are advocating for. Why not use this to our advantage?)[3]

Baby steps are okay.

Still, there should be lines when it comes to picking and choosing how we project our confidence. Because you know what confidence definitely *doesn't* look like? Basking in our insecurities and self-doubts, ruminating over past mistakes, and never giving ourselves breaks.

Confidence requires holding oneself accountable and taking action to unlearn bad habits, as well as internal maintenance to keep the foundation of our confidence stable and resilient. It is not something one "chooses" to possess and then suddenly has. One must act, exert oneself, and take risks. We each have what it takes, regardless of the ways the Effortless Perfection Myth may try to convince us we do not. It's time to start building our confidence higher and applauding other women working toward the same goal.

Section III

Reclaiming What's Ours

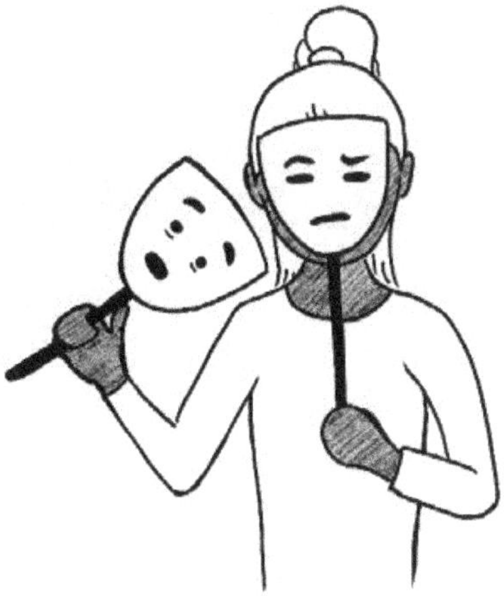

Chapter 15

Is There Any Right Way for a Woman to Be Assertive?

MY FAVORITE PROTEST SIGN at the 2016 Women's March read: "I know. I know. I'm standing up for myself. I'm such a bitch." In my mind, this statement highlights the impossible double-bind women face when trying to come across as both assertive and likeable. We want to believe that we as a society have grown more comfortable with women showing strength and wielding power, but when it comes down to it, assertive behavior still elicits different emotional responses depending on the gender of the person performing the behavior.

Undeniably, we've been conditioned to value men and women according to different standards—standards based off what traditional gender roles and stereotypes tell us we should expect from each other. The famous Heidi-Howard study demonstrates this. Two Harvard professors wrote a case study about real-life entrepreneur Heidi Roizen, describing how she had used her professional network and outgoing personality to succeed as a venture capitalist. Half their class read the case study with Heidi's real name at the top and the other half read a case study that was identical except that the first name had been changed to "Howard." When asked to rate the two, students felt both were equally skilled, but thought Howard seemed "determined, driven, someone you'd want to work for," while Heidi seemed "selfish, bossy, not someone you'd want to work for."[1]

Gender determined the likability of these two candidates because we judge people according to preexisting stereotypes: Women are supposed to be communitarian (less personally assertive), whereas men are allowed to be more individualistic (more personally assertive).[2] So even if women wanted to be able to act in ways that more forcibly advance their interests and demonstrate their ability to be insistent and decisive, doing so would engender pushback that could hurt their social standing. It's a classic "damned if you do, damned if you don't" scenario.

To make matters even more complicated, the Effortless Perfection Myth comes along and throws itself into the mix with its own insane demands: *One or the other is not going to cut it. The Effortlessly Perfect women has to find a way to be all things to all people. Make it work.* Consequently, many of us do our best to avoid situations that might force us to make the decision between being assertive and being likeable; we particularly dislike negotiation.

In their book *Women Don't Ask,* Linda Babcock and Sara Laschever note a major difference in the way men and women view negotiation. Apparently, men tend to see situations involving debate and bargaining as opportunities for gain that could even potentially be fun, while women tend to see these same situations more as traps to be avoided at all costs.

Furthermore, we don't always see the point in engaging to begin with. Babcock and Laschever discuss what they refer to as a "turnip-to-oyster" scale derived from the opposing axioms "you can't get blood from a turnip" and "the world is your oyster."[3] The turnip position on the scale belongs to individuals who experience the world as being controlled primarily by outside forces, making them believe that their environments are essentially unchangeable. By contrast, the oyster position belongs to individuals who experience the world as primarily controlled by internal forces, bringing them to see their environments as adaptable and capable of meeting their needs and desires by allowing them to have a hand in the outcomes. Guess which category women are

45 percent more likely to fall under?[4]

That's right—Team Turnip. Women tend to operate according to the perception that their circumstances are more fixed and absolute than they really are, and that someone or something else is in control. Babcock and Laschever explicate, "This assumption—the result of powerful social influences that go to work the day a woman is born—has a broad impact on women's behavior. Instead of looking for ways to improve a difficult situation, women often assume that they are 'stuck' with their circumstances."[5]

No wonder women don't tend to assert themselves or negotiate for things they want. They do not fully believe that their efforts can actually alter their circumstances. As Alice Walker says, "The most common way people give up their power is by thinking they don't have any." She is speaking to us!

What does all of this stuff about agency, assertiveness, and control have to do with the seductive power of the Effortless Perfection Myth? Easy. When we abide by the Effortless Perfection Myth, we are really just attempting to reclaim the control we feel is so far out of our hands. The train of thought goes: *If I can't have agency within my environment, if outside forces are what decide my fate and my future, then my best bet is to make myself as close as I can into the image that those external forces expect and demand from me. If I can win their favor (never mind who "their" is alluding to), I will feel more in control of my life and more confident that things will go the way I hope and intend.*

Unfortunately, instead of gaining control through Effortless Perfection, we often relinquish even more power to it. Because we receive a mini-confidence boost each time we live up to its standards, we are led to develop self-confidence built on fleeting, conditional moments. The stronger our reliance on these boosts, the greater our reassurance addiction to external approval grows, and the more entrapped we become within the Myth.

In this way, the Effortless Perfection Myth derives much of its strength from accompanying social sanctions, or "social reaction[s] of approval or disapproval in response to someone's actions" which then regulate and enforce a "standard of behavior that is deemed socially acceptable."[6] Whether a verbal response, facial expression, or passage of judgment, we pay attention to the reactions elicited from others every time we say or do something. Consideration of what others will think of us if we do XYZ action becomes an automatic part of one's decision-making process, leading this social system of reward and punishment to become internalized and reflected in our day-to-day behavior.

As a result of social sanctions, we collectively impose and enforce the status quo on each other. This system of social control has positive aspects. It plays a huge role in keeping people from stealing, lying, and other decidedly immoral things because they know others will respond with condemning social sanctions if they do. But the system also has negative aspects. It can keep people from being true to themselves and their desires by leading them to internalize a value system like Effortless Perfection without second thought, instead of coming to a personalized value system on their own terms.

My understanding of social sanctions is a big reason why I get frustrated when things like self-sacrifice, fear of confrontation, and inability to be assertive are labeled as inherently female, self-imposed handicaps. This behavior is not part of our genetic code; it is learned via gendered socialization wherein we were rewarded for exhibiting and punished for contradicting traditional gender roles over the course of our lives.

Why does so much of the advice given to women about boosting our confidence and claiming space put the onus entirely on us, as though the timidity we feel when negotiating or the tremor that enters our voice when trying to stand up for ourselves is nobody's fault but our own? *Why aren't we considering the possibility that women have a hard time asserting themselves because there still does not exist a way for us to be assertive without receiving negative social sanctions as retribution?*

How are we supposed to be self-confident and decisive without worrying others will consciously or subconsciously judge us? This was a major concern for my interviewees, most of whom often felt the need to minimize and apologize for their intelligence, beauty, and talent so as to seem less threatening.

Some even noted performing inadvertent acts of self-sabotage when trying to come across as serious and strong. One mentioned that, when delivering difficult news or confronting someone who has wronged her, she gesticulates in an exaggerated, almost goofy manner to distract from the harsher, unhumorous tone of her words. Another discussed commonly finding herself speaking decisively and then immediately following up with an apology to "ease up on the intensity or perceived demanding-ness" of the interaction. For instance, she might say, "Sorry, does that make sense?" after delivering a directive.

I bonded with several of my interviewees over the frustration of crying when angry—a habit that infuriates me to no end because it completely switches the tone of the interaction and the meaning of my words, when all I want is to come across as strong and resolute.

I never questioned this tendency until attending a book talk for Rebecca Traister's *Good and Mad: The Revolutionary Power of Women's Anger.* She pointed out that many women, particularly white women, express their anger in the form of tears because it allows us to let out our frustration in a way that has been deemed less threatening and more socially appropriate. Tears equate to sadness and vulnerability, and that fragility plays more neatly into rigid gender norms that like to cast women as damsels in distress.

For instance, it is harder for my male partner to respond to my anger with anger if I am crying. Tears inspire empathy that straight-up anger does not. This could certainly be considered a form of emotional manipulation on my part were it intentional, but it's not. I just think that, somewhere deep down, my body knows that female displays of anger and assertiveness are not typically well-received, so my reaction cloaks itself in sadness to make itself more "palatable."

I don't like the way societal assumptions about what constitutes appropriate female behavior act as a kind of "psychological straitjacket" restraining my ability to be forward with my emotions.[7] I want to be more honest with myself and those I love. So much of what constitutes being Effortlessly Perfect women bars us from sharing our full truth with others. It is more than an attack on our mental health; it is an attack on our integrity.

We've been mistaken to believe our tears always come from a place of sadness. Sometimes they are actually gasoline begging for a flame.[8] So light a match, ladies—it's time to burn this Myth and all its godforsaken gender traps to the ground.

Chapter 16

The Seductive Power of Niceness and Unanimity

AS SOMEONE WHO WAS LONG DEDICATED to upholding the "good girl" persona required by Effortless Perfection, it took me until late in my junior year to realize that I was not required to pretend I agreed with everything that was said to me or to go along with nearly every situation I found myself in the midst of even if I wasn't entirely on board. The concept of saying "no" and not needing to give a ten-minute explanation-apology was pretty foreign to me. It took me even longer to realize that it was okay to have strong opinions and not apologize for them, since I'd grown so used to shying away from conflict.

Gloria Steinem refers to this form of silencing as the "seductive power of niceness and unanimity."[1] The phrase alludes to the way in which it can be tempting in situations of possible discord to just go with the flow and not draw attention to oneself, especially when going against the grain can feel particularly uncomfortable for women. "I have trouble calling people out because I always want to be on everyone's good side," notes Mia.

Conversely, Jordan used to beat herself up for her inability to keep her strong feelings and opinions to herself. "I used to think to myself, my life would be so much easier if I could just learn how to shut up and not speak my mind," she says. She agonized over what she felt was a "personal problem" until she realized that feeling inclined to speak up for herself actually put her ahead of the game. She reclaimed her voice as a source of power and watched as other women struggled to unlearn the "seductive power of niceness and unanimity" that had never fully caught on for her.

Others have had to expend much more energy breaking this habit. Laura attests to how inviting "the path of least resistance" can be in situations where not everyone in the room shares her political beliefs:

> *I have to calibrate how strongly I want to respond. Is it worth it to explain three times at one dinner party that a certain female political figure isn't a "witch"? Or to get mad at my brother for saying something is "so gay," something that deeply upsets me, even when I know he won't change his behavior? Sometimes I deal with it and sometimes I decide to just smile and nod. Sometimes that makes me feel sick afterwards, other times it makes me feel exhausted. I'm hyperaware of my inclination toward yessing people and how attuned I am to self-correcting based on the company, and how I do it a lot more than my male family members and friends.*

Laura's awareness of her inclinations to "self-correct" in addition to her ability to check in with herself to decide whether she has it in her in the moment to stand up and say something is admirable. That kind of calculation allows for self-care, which in turn serves as a great defense against burnout.

That said, Laura is also quick to point out that there is a balance that must be met to make sure we are still upholding our values. We need to be cognizant of when it's really not worth speaking up versus when it's just the "seductive power of niceness and unanimity" coaxing us into silence. For many women, it can be hard to act on our beliefs, no matter how strong, if we feel like they might not be 100 percent well-received. If there's even *just one* person in the crowd we think will be dismayed, we feel pressure to pull back.

Blake offers insight that part of our motivation for staying quiet could be influenced by the desire to play the part of the "chill girl" in our social circles, who has mastered effortlessness by always appearing a perfect mix of amiable and indifferent. Her "unbothered" and "at ease" nature allows her to come across as "chill," regardless of the situation.

Blake references a *Vogue* article that captures the way she feels expected to act as an undergrad. The piece's author, Martine Thompson, talks about a period in her life during which she tried to become the "most chill, fabulously blasé person ever," only to find that it led her to "an elusive halfway point between a desensitized robot and a whimsical movie character, a functioning fragment of [herself] perennially unfazed by everyone and everything, convinced this would somehow improve [her] life."[2] She advises that pretending to be unfazed in all situations all the time is not a good strategy for reaching life fulfillment—even if it's what Effortless Perfection tells us will make us the most likeable and popular.

The main issue Thompson ran into was that, because she felt the need always to act like she didn't care either way, she found herself in a very unhealthy state of mind. She satirizes, "You've done something wildly offensive I'll be overanalyzing for days…months…years? No worries, it's chill! I've invested in you, and you're still dodging commitment like it's your national sport? It's chill; far be it from me to enforce boundaries where my self-worth and general wellness are prioritized."[3] The article further emphasizes how being "the chill girl" requires always watching oneself "through the lens of others," acting as a social chameleon contorting oneself into something more "palatable" for the next person.

We need to recognize that, in committing ourselves to being effortlessly "chill," we are essentially giving up our backbones. We are devaluing our feelings and emotions, which means devaluing ourselves by extension. I don't think those of us in college striving for the "cool/chill girl" award realize how much we are giving up by doing so. Thompson concludes her article by highlighting how prone to manipulation this way of being made her and calls out the "cultural need to pathologize women" who are willing to speak their minds and forge their own non-whimsical identities.[4]

The moral of the story? It's okay to take up space. Our opinions and experiences as women are allowed to hold more than a little weight. We needn't shrink ourselves in order not to bump up against others' beliefs. We don't have to ask permission to have our needs considered. We are allowed to make self-care a priority without being considered selfish.

Coming to these enlightening realizations takes a good deal of time and work. Women must grapple with the older instincts and impulses blocking us from doing so. We have to *un*learn part of our socialization through the process of questioning things that have always seemed implicit.

In college, my friend Daniella always seemed to be one step ahead of me on this journey, probably because she learned much earlier on than I did that unnecessary apologies and explanations were encumbrances she could do without. Far from making her judgmental or close-minded, this approach quickly enabled her to become a widely respected role model whom countless students on campus looked up to and went to for advice. Better yet, she was never shy about using her clout to bring attention to numerous social justice issues on campus. She is pictured on the next page in a poster for the Who Needs Feminism Campaign.

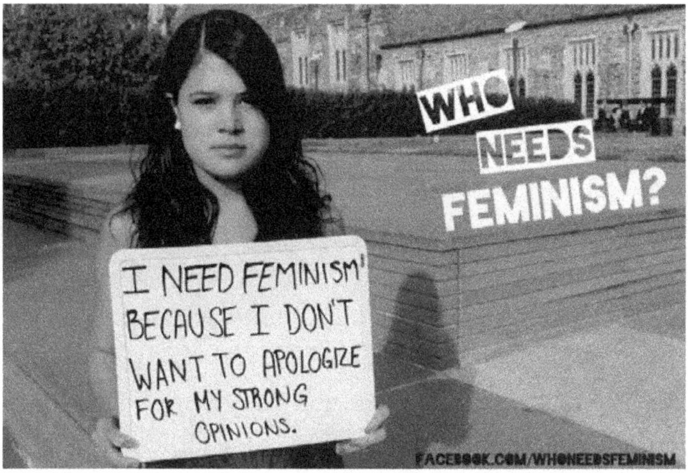

[5]

This PR campaign for feminism was launched at Duke our sophomore year and has since spread far and wide to campuses across the country and beyond. Its aims are to combat how feminism is "both misunderstood and denigrated regularly on a broad societal scale" by highlighting all the movement has done and promises to do for us.[6] *Check it out at whoneedsfeminism.tumblr.com.*

Total badass, right? The first time I saw this poster on one of the bulletin boards in the student center, I was in such awe. I remember thinking, *Wow, it would take so much more courage and confidence than I possess to be able to lend my name and face to such an assertive message, especially knowing it would be posted all around campus for everyone to see.* Having already begun my journey into the world of gender issues, I no doubt identified with the feminist movement, but to claim it in the way Daniella had with such a strong fervor…well, at the time it just seemed too scary.[i]

[i] Daniella was kind enough to look over one of my early book drafts, and the best part of this is that she left me the following note: "This is funny to read because OF COURSE I thought and worried about the same things. I think we are so quick to attribute self-assurance to other women, but so resistant to adopt it for ourselves. Luckily, I do think I have a lot of self-assurance now. At that moment, though, it was more a leap of faith. Support from friends like you fueled me forward!" This is why we need friends who back us and our values. It can feel scary to act on behalf of those values in a public way, but when you have a strong community behind you it gives you the strength to do what needs to be done.

I was intimidated by the potential social sanctions I might receive if I were to do the same thing. I worried people might label me as overly dogmatic, unable to take a joke, a bra-burning man-hater (ugh, that forsaken stereotype). I worried potential romantic interests might be turned off, that guy friends and maybe even girl friends would disapprove. All these thoughts and fears I felt intensely upon seeing this powerful image of Daniella.

Yet all those feelings compounded didn't even hold a candle to the flush of disappointment I felt in myself. I wanted to be able to take the same kind of action. I wanted to be able to own my beliefs and trust in my experiences in the same way. But my "good girl" hardwiring, courtesy of the Effortless Perfection Myth, still had me backed into a corner. *I couldn't possibly pull off something like that,* I thought to myself. *I want to, but…just…no.*

Lucky for me, I still had time to come around. Also lucky for me, I had friends like Daniella and other mentors on campus to act as strong influencers in getting me to the places I wanted to go. Funny how much can change in a year or two. Today, having a poster statement like Daniella's with my name and face on it seems so easy and obvious, but only because I've had time to grow into my feminist beliefs and feel the benefits for myself. I've come to see that, for the occasional negative social sanction I may receive for this kind of expression, there is always a plethora of positive ones, from both women and men. I've seen how those who look up to me as a mentor and older role model receive additional benefit when I take a stand because it allows them to feel more confident and comfortable expressing themselves in similar ways.

The first step, for me, was realizing that such empowerment does not and cannot result from avoiding conflict altogether, all the time. It comes from raising your voice when things move you to do so, from making a point you feel passionate about and not following it up with a series of unnecessary justifiers. It takes time to *un*learn conflict as something to fear and, instead, to *re*learn conflict as something that is okay and sometimes even necessary.

Chapter 17

Anger Doesn't Always Have to Be a Bad Thing

"ANGER IS SOMETHING I've always felt is wrong, that in expressing it you are making it seem like something is wrong with you, you are out of control," Jordan tells me. Her opinion mirrors the majority response of the young women whom I interviewed, though she gives my favorite depiction of actually dealing with these kinds of feelings. The personal process she has adopted for analyzing the validity of her anger and deciding whether to express it feels somewhat ridiculous (in a way that makes you inclined to laugh), while still all too familiar (in a way that makes you laugh more at yourself than anything else).

Like most women, Jordan often feels the need to jump through hoops before opening her mouth to express negative emotions:

> *Particularly in relationships, so say I'm angry at my boyfriend, I have to check with my girlfriends in a text or call like, "I'm so angry with him! Is this just me? Should I express this or not?" And then I'll explain the situation to like four people and I'm like, "Do I have a right to be angry? Okay, I do?! Okay, now I'm gonna go spend 30 minutes crafting this text explaining why I'm angry and then I'm gonna send it back to you, you are going to read the text, and we are going to figure out if I'm coming off as the right amount of angry or if I sound psycho and then I can send it."*

Jordan's checklist for validating both her anger and her expression of it is extensive because female anger is received differently than male anger.

In fact, studies show that when a man expresses anger during a debate, those listening are more likely to consider his argument and abandon their original position on the matter, whereas when a woman expresses anger during a debate, the opposite response typically occurs. This holds true even when women don't realize that their assertiveness is being registered by others as anger.[1]

Jordan laments, "Guys can be like, 'I have this emotion and I have these three options of how to act it out.' But for girls, it's like 'I have this emotion, it's wrong.'" It feels wrong because expressing it may cause conflict, and conflict is a sign that she is not successfully playing the role of the Effortlessly Perfect, "easy to love," "chill" chick.

Even when women do feel somewhat comfortable expressing that they are less than thrilled about something, we still feel the need to do so carefully. Tone and wording must be carefully chosen. Julie explains, "The expectations in terms of disagreement are just different for men and women. We are seen as antagonistic when we are only voicing a differing thought, while I've seen men *actually* be antagonistic and not be labeled that way." It's hard to not to let such judgments sway us from using our voices.

Abby additionally muses, "Say I get frustrated at the same thing a man gets frustrated at, and I'm expressing the same thing, in pretty much the same way—why am I viewed as 'emotional' and 'bitchy,' when he's just seen as 'angry' and that's it?" She's right to be upset. These three adjectives may pop up as synonyms in a thesaurus, but they each carry a nuanced definition dependent upon connotation.

The word "emotional" not so secretly links to the stereotype that women are hormonal and our feelings too often get the best of us, while "bitchy" is a word engineered to refer to women in a demeaning manner, with no real male equivalent. Both are coded pejoratives. They are words that hold implicit meanings that reinforce sexism, even if in a discreet manner. "Angry," on the other hand, is not a gendered word and has a pretty straightforward meaning, so men get the benefit of the noncoded adjective in this situation. We aren't afforded the same privilege.

This rings particularly true for women of color. Lily from Duke discusses the added implications of expressing dissent as an African American woman who all too often faces the risk of being labeled the "Angry Black Woman." She notes, "Voicing that you disagree or have a different perspective is more likely to be interpreted as threatening or volatile when coming from a Black woman. It's unfair, but it's true."

Furthermore, in part because of the way their concerns often get written off as part of this biased caricature, "it feels like the cause of [Black women's] anger is never investigated... like whatever is upsetting us, it just doesn't matter because we are 'overreacting' anyway." Such apathetic sentiments contribute to the intense pressures Black women feel, not only to avoid coming off as "too angry," but also to appear strong and stoic all the time, as if the issues they face don't impact them as much as they actually do.

The overall expectation is that Black women are able to "do anything, take anything," explains Lily. "Now, obviously Black women are strong. But on an individual basis, we are also human. Everyone needs space to be vulnerable, to mess up, to come into their own. You can't do that unless you are given space to grow and have reckless abandon about you. Black women are not afforded that by the larger community or their own community." While Lily feels that parts of the medical world are beginning to connect the dots that "expecting women to always appear strong creates added stressors that can and have led to development of serious mental and physical health issues," she also believes there is a long way to go.

It is worth recognizing that if young women under the influence of Effortless Perfection culture feel pressure to pretend everything is going well all the time in their lives, women of color often feel it doubly so. They feel pressure to live up to their campus community's standard of perfection, as well as pressure from their racial community to be a particular kind of strong. We need to keep this in mind when pushing back against this harmful status quo.

Because of the different ways we tend to struggle with negative feelings, most women, not so shockingly, find it easier to compartmentalize them rather than to speak them out loud. Mia and Jane both express feeling that the only times they are willing to put their anger "out there" is when venting to people they know very, very well, such as their parents or their closest friend. "It's like, I'm not losing you [if I express this]. It's okay," says Mia.

Jane affirms, "I definitely feel like I can't just freak out to anybody. It has to be someone who understands me and isn't going to judge me for the things I'm mad about." For these women and many more, anger is an embarrassing emotion that can be hard to reveal to even our most trusted confidants, let alone the person causing our distress.

In her book *The Nice Girl Syndrome*, Beverly Engel provides reasons women don't tend to express anger outright, which not so shockingly include fear of retaliation and being labeled negatively. "We fear that expressing anger will deny the nurturing aspects of women's socialization or drive away the love and closeness women seek," she notes.[2] (There are those social sanctions at play again, saying: *Nuh-uh-uh, Effortless Perfection and anger can't live in the same body.*)

But anger doesn't necessarily have to be a bad thing. From a biological stance, anger can be a very good thing; it is simply "a stress response to internal or external demands, threats or pressure."[3] When anger wells up inside, that feeling of alertness and reactivity is functioning both as a warning system and a survival mechanism. Anger can be used to reveal to us how much we care about or are impacted by something. It makes us viscerally aware of when emotional issues need to be addressed, expectations are not being met, and relational ties are forcing us to compromise too many of our beliefs and values. From there, anger can motivate us to make changes and to reinforce our boundaries by catalyzing us to stand up for ourselves.

Despite all these benefits, many women are socialized to deny their own natural expression of anger. We are taught that anger is bad, and for us to feel it makes us bad. But this only harms us further because, even though we aren't directly expressing our anger, it does not miraculously go away. Suppressing our emotions is not the same as eliminating them. Engel explains:

> *Each emotion has a purpose, and that emotion will remain with you, buried inside your body, locked up in your psyche, until that purpose is recognized and understood...it is also important to realize that as long as you are angry, you will exude a certain kind of angry energy. Sometimes this energy is palpable and is consciously experienced by others. Other times, it is felt only subliminally by others, but is felt nonetheless. People are affected by your anger whether it is overt or not and whether they are aware of it or not. They will respond by getting angry along with you, by acting your anger out for you, or by being on guard around you.*[4]

Our fear of anger and conflict is often what stokes the fire for exactly that—anger and conflict. Instead of a series of small bonfire-size blazes, easily controlled and extinguished once the causes are identified, we allow our emotional forests to dry and dry until one spark sets the whole thing aflame into a huge, unpredictable wildfire. By not expressing anger, we become resentful; we hold it in and deny it, eventually displacing it on those who don't really deserve it (or at least not all of it).

As my mentor Gary Glass once said to me, "Conflict is a way of strengthening the relationships that actually matter to us." If you aren't bringing up something that's impacting your connection with another—whether because you fear the discomfort it may bring or you just don't want to make the effort—there is a greater problem at hand. The mark of a healthy relationship is not lack of argument and conflict; it's the way two people communicate when such problems arise. Anger is not what leads to hurt—it's what we do with that anger, how we choose to express that anger.

Our ability to channel our anger in order to assertively say what we need and want in our relationships is one of the key things that allow us to be intimately vulnerable with our loved ones in the first place. "One of the greatest (and least discussed) barriers to compassion practice is fear of setting boundaries and holding people accountable," writes Brené Brown.[5] The better we are at accepting ourselves and others, the more compassionate we become, but "it's difficult to accept people when they are hurting us or taking advantage of us or walking all over us."[6]

That's where boundaries and accountability come into play. By assertively setting personal boundaries and holding people accountable when they cross them (whether or not they knew they were doing so at the time), we create an environment wherein we are freer to show kindness and vulnerability and compassion because we have our own set of positive self-protection mechanisms in place. By being "kinder, but firmer," we open ourselves up to relationships of greater love, intimacy, and understanding.[7] And that's why so many of us are chasing after Effortless Perfection in the first place, right? To feel worthy of love?

Chapter 18
#NoApologies

IF ASSERTIVENESS IS IMPORTANT not only in protecting ourselves but in making our relationships stronger, how can we more fully integrate it into our daily lives? Perhaps we could begin with issues as simple as upspeak and over-apologizing.

Upspeak is the female tendency to heighten our pitch as we near the end of sentences, causing our statements to sound more like apologetic questions. Tina Fey humorously advises against this behavior in her book *Bossypants*: "No one wants to go to a doctor who says, 'I'm going to be your surgeon? I'm here to talk to you about your procedure? I was first in my class at Johns Hopkins, so?'"[1] We must pay attention to how we deliver our opinions and ideas. We need to consider whether we are truly delivering our statements *as statements*.

Furthermore, we need to consider the way we employ the symbolic word "sorry" in everyday situations that don't really require apology. Sloane Crosley of the *New York Times* observes, "For so many women…apologies are inexorably linked with our conception of politeness. Somehow, as we grew into adults, 'sorry' became an entry point to basic affirmative sentences."[2] (You know the whole "Hey! Sorry! I was just wondering…")

Huffington Post journalist Ani Vrabel additionally points out that the word "sorry" isn't really an appropriate synonym for "I have a question" or "I didn't see you there and you startled me!" or "Allow me to move out of the way." It is best saved for situations where one wishes to convey, "I made a poor decision or did something wrong and it impacted you negatively. I recognize this and feel bad about it and would like to make things better between us."[3] To use a word that carries those kinds of apologetic connotations in such frequent everyday situations weakens the meaning of the word "sorry."

The habit of overapologizing is linked to Effortless Perfection because we feel pressure to be a "chill girl" who welcomes the "seductive power of niceness and unanimity." Effortless Perfection tell us it's better to apologize, take the blame, and eliminate any possibility for conflict. This is supposed to make us "easy to love," but is the love we theoretically recieve in exchange really worth the price being paid?

Over-apologizing weakens our ability to tell others how we really feel, sometimes even detracting from our expressions of gratitude for one another. For example, when we are feeling down about ourselves, we sometimes substitute in the word "sorry" when we really mean to use the words "thank you." Comic artist Yao Xiao demonstrates this in one of her pieces wherein she depicts a series of characters in juxtaposed scenarios under headlines of: "If you want to say ______, don't say ______."[4] Some scenarios include:

- If you want to say, "Thank you for listening," don't say, "Sorry I'm just rambling."
- If you want to say, "Thank you for spending time with me," don't say, "Sorry I'm kind of a drag."
- If you want to say, "Thank you for having hope in me this whole time," don't say, "Sorry I'm such a disappointment."

This way, we can make sure to appreciate others for what they have done without seeming to knock on ourselves. We come off as stronger *and* more sincere.

In 2014, the Baldwin Scholars program[i] at Duke put together the #NoApologies Campaign, encouraging undergrad women to recognize self-defeating internalized habits and mindsets imposed by gender norms, such as apologizing unnecessarily—hence the name and hashtag. The campaign sought to provide tangible tools to address how these habits and mindsets play a role in our everyday lives.

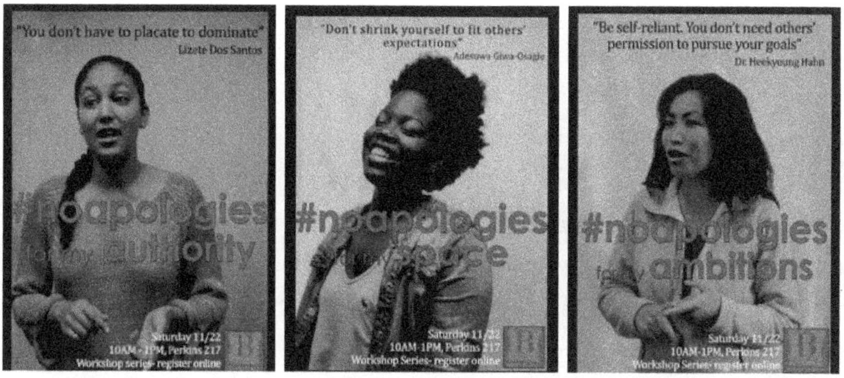

5, 6, 7

A #NoApologies workshop was promoted by a series of motivational posters across campus. Each inspirational image pictured a female student or faculty leader along with a personally crafted statement in line with the campaign's theme.

---

[i] This program, meant to "inspire and support female-identified undergraduate students to become engaged, confident and connected leaders in the Duke community and beyond," was created in response to the findings of the Duke Women's Initiative Report—the same report that coined the term "Effortless Perfection." It is a great example of programming that institutions of higher learning could be investing in to empower female undergrads and push back against the Myth. Find out more at www.baldwinscholars.duke.edu/program.

Seeing these posters of strong female leaders all across campus was incredibly empowering, as I had yet to see such a subtle but pervasive women's issue addressed during my time in college. Just the name for the campaign—#NoApologies—made such a poignant statement. It was and has been exciting to witness awareness being brought to these kinds of issues both on and off college campuses.

Beyond the Baldwin Scholars, national advertisers have recently begun catching on to the reemerging trend of "girl power." One such ad that has received a great deal of attention is Pantene's commercial "Not Sorry."[8] It begins with a series of shots demonstrating how women slip "sorry" into sentences in the same way tweens use the word "like"—almost as a reflex. One shot occurs in a corporate boardroom with a woman at the table interjecting, "Sorry, can I ask a stupid question?" Another shot has a woman opening a door to ask a fellow employee, "Sorry, do you have a minute?" The issue being addressed is subtle. The commercial is observing how apologizing unnecessarily is typical female behavior, and makes the audience think about what that means on a deeper level.

Halfway through the commercial, a white screen with the simple phrase "Don't be sorry" pops up, leading into the second half of the video. This time around the same women are in the same scenarios, but employ different wordings that work just as well, if not better, than "sorry."

The first woman smoothly says, "I have a question" and seamlessly dives into her point, without weakening her statement by using an unnecessary qualifier. The next one opts for "Morning. You got a minute?" Notice that these scenarios involve only slightly altered reactions. The ad isn't calling for women to take it upon themselves to stand up on the spot and give long remarks about the prevalence of subtle sexism, it's simply giving examples of possible changes that could emerge from a little extra awareness.

After all, apologizing all the time is just another way of reinforcing the gendered stereotype that women can't be as assertive. We should recognize our habit of apologizing incessantly for what it is—a form of internalized sexism that we need to kick. It takes time to unlearn what we as women have been taught to be sorry for, but it is one of the first steps toward reclaiming what is ours—space, time, agency, respect.

As a quick aside: if you read this chapter and though to yourself, "Ugh. That is so me," I recommend checking out a Chrome app called the Just Not Sorry extension. This app helps its users to stop using words like "just" and "sorry," as well as phrases like "I'm no expert" and "Does that make sense?" in our emails by underlining them in red like a common typo. These words and phrases are qualifiers that inadvertently minimize others' confidence in our ideas by "clutter[ing] up [our] emails, undermin[ing our] authority, and dilut[ing our] leadership capacity," notes *Slate* writer Christina Cauterucci.[9] We don't need that! The small reminder provided by this app is a great way to begin realigning our subconscious word choices toward something more effective and powerful.

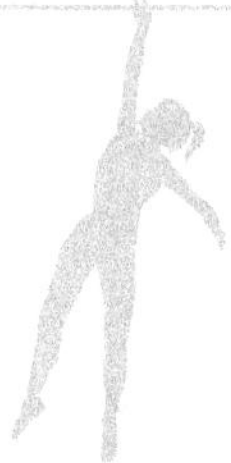

Chapter 19

The Dubious Partnership Between Lack of Healthy Entitlement and Need for Validation

ENTITLEMENT IS one of my least favorite words. I hate the arrogant, spoiled connotations associated with it. And yet a quick Google search pulls up synonyms like "free," "at liberty," "allowed," "permitted," "unrestricted," and "unconstrained." Entitlement, I have come to see, can be a good thing—as long as it is kept at a *healthy* bay.

If you don't feel comfortable with the idea that there are things you deserve—something I now understand is *necessary* for getting to a place of "Enough"—it is definitely something to work on. The Effortless Perfection Myth keeps us chasing its hollow trophy by convincing us we must always be proving we have worth and have earned the right to love and respect, when such things should really be inherent. We should feel entitled to love and respect, regardless.

Women's low sense of personal entitlement is one of the greatest obstacles holding us back. Before we can demand better, we have to first believe that we deserve better or, at the very least, that we deserve to be able to *ask* for better, without feeling guilty or apologetic. Until we do so, women will go on expecting smaller rewards for the work we do and feeling the need to work harder for the rewards we get.[1] The wage gap will continue, the lack of women in politics and top-ranked positions of authority will remain, imposter syndrome will rage on—you get the picture.

And, yes, in case you were wondering, it really is true that women expect smaller rewards for the work we do and feel the need to work harder for the rewards we get. This trend has been demonstrated time after time through numerous studies. In one such study, psychologists Charlene Callahan-Levy and Lawrence Messe recruited college students to write a series of opinion pieces about campus-related issues. While doing so, half were told to decide how much money to pay themselves for doing the task and half were told to decide how much to pay other participants for the task. The researchers found that women paid themselves an average of 19 percent less than males paid themselves. Women also paid others (including other women) more than they paid themselves, a trend that was not found among the men.[2]

Furthermore, participant evaluations showed no gender differences in how well students performed the tasks, suggesting that when asked to pay themselves it was as if women "simply lost their abilities to accurately evaluate what the work was worth when they were the ones performing the task."[3] This demonstrates how "many women wait to be rewarded for their efforts…because they don't know whether they deserve something unless someone else tells them that they do."[4] Think of the implications of this, of not knowing whether we deserve something unless some outside power tells us we do! This is no doubt our reassurance addictions kicking in. Thanks to the Effortless Perfection Myth and the way it guts us of even the slightest sense of healthy entitlement, we are unprepared to take full advantage of our talents and improve our lives!

In a similar study on entitlement, participants were told to perform a task until they had "earned" four dollars. Unobserved, women worked 22 percent longer than the men. When monitored by an experimenter, women worked a whopping 52 percent longer, while the men worked roughly the same amount whether unobserved or observed. Not only do these findings show us that women feel less entitled to the earnings of their work, but it "tells us that women have learned that they must pay more attention than men to the impression they make on others, presumably because they fear the penalties for counter-stereotypical behavior."[5] Incredibly eye-opening.

Interviewees Melissa and Piper mentioned multiple experiences in their STEM classes and labs that paralleled the trends demonstrated by these studies. "In CompSci class, some guys will be on their phones and are just more likely to mess around," Melissa says. "I think girls just have more of an awareness like they are being watched at all times."

Piper additionally notes: "In BioChem labs, I've noticed guys are usually a bit more messy and rushed, while the girls I've worked alongside are all like me where we feel like we need to be meticulous and cover all bases. We need to deserve this. We need to know every detail of it." Obviously, it's never good to generalize entirely, but in these two scenarios it appears that the standard the female students feel intense pressure to pursue is Effortless Perfection, while evidently the male students' standard is simply "good enough."

Men seem to come into the classroom, STEM classrooms in particular, with a greater sense of belonging there, which is likely linked to a sense of conscious or subconscious entitlement that they are deserving of being in that space. Women seem to have a harder time grasping onto that sense of deserving to be there, too.

From where exactly does this lack of healthy entitlement in females spring? John Jost, an assistant professor of organizational behavior at Yale, calls the phenomenon "depressed-entitlement effect" and affirms it appears in much greater measure among women.[6] If unchecked, this propensity to undermine our self-esteem, our confidence, and our assertiveness will continue to rob us of what we deserve. We must come to terms with the fact that a bit of entitlement doesn't have to be a bad thing because not to have any entitlement at all is to believe we deserve nothing. And I'm really, *really* not okay with that. We can and should be wary of entitlement, but we are not allowed to swear it off altogether.

Lack of healthy entitlement and the need for outside validation go hand in hand. Both are inextricably spun into the Effortless Perfection Myth, because lack of entitlement, of feeling like we must constantly work to prove we deserve basic courtesies like respect and kindness, is what fuels the reassurance addictions that require outside forces to approve of us before we are able to approve of ourselves.

British-Afghan writer Mohadesa Najumi elegantly argues in her viral article "Why the Woman Who Does Not Require Validation from Anyone Is the Most Feared Individual on the Planet" that the moment a woman rejects the need for validation, she becomes a much more powerful threat to the status quo and, thus, a greater force with which to be reckoned.[7] She does not need someone else to tell her who she is or what she deserves; she can do that on her own. By not allowing herself to take too much stock in society's perception of her, she is free to forge her own image and more empowered to act against societal expectations that might otherwise hold her back.

I've chosen to end this chapter (and section of the book focused on assertiveness) with a series of anecdotes from college wherein I learned, over and over, how to best handle my inclinations to reach out for validation, as the Effortless Perfection Myth had long socialized me to do. I think they are important to share because they provide concrete examples of how college-aged women can push back against inclinations to seek validation and, instead, feel entitled to a sense of self-assuredness.

Anecdote 1: I wasn't the biggest drinker during my first two years of college. I already had a great deal of energy and outgoingness and never really felt I needed a social lubricant to get that part of me active. Still, whenever I was pressured to drink, I always felt required to give some long excuse as to why I couldn't, as opposed to just a "no thanks." The thing with these kinds of excuses is that they are pretty easy to see through. When others see you feel the need to make such excuses, it becomes clear that you care more than just a little about their stance on the matter, too. They become aware that you are worried about how they are perceiving you, which then gives them the ability to flex that power if they so choose, only making you more susceptible to peer pressure.

The truth is I never needed to give an excuse, I just needed to be resolute. The secret here is this: *How you see yourself and your decisions impacts how others ultimately see you and your decisions. If you present both in a way that shows you aren't hungry for validation because you don't have a starving need for approval begging to be fed, others are more likely to hold that decision of yours in high regard without challenging it.*

Anecdote 2: When I first declared women's studies as a second major, I wasn't always comfortable talking about it. When people asked what I studied, there were plenty of times I would just say public policy, and leave it at that. In the times I didn't choose to omit my second major entirely, it would often come with a long explanation, a thinly veiled version of: "… and women's studies, *but it's not what you think….*" Regardless of how happy I was with my decision, I still felt the need to make others approve of it. And here's the thing, just like with the drinking, it's one thing to make a statement and move on; people don't really tend to question as much that way because you give them less space to do so. But if you present it with a follow-up string of justifications, that space grows.

I'd embraced feminism and women's studies because of the empowering beliefs it instilled in me: I was allowed to take up more space, my opinions mattered, and I needn't feel guilty for wanting the things I wanted or ashamed for doing the things I was doing outside "normalized" gendered tropes. How ironic that I still felt the decision to study this topic required such extensive backpedaling and justification.

The secret here is this: *You can't allow the pieces at the heart of your identity, the thoughts and beliefs most valuable to you, to be invalidated by the opinions of others who have never taken the time to truly consider those same things in the same way.*

Anecdote 3: My final semester, I got a tattoo. At twenty-two, after a long period of consideration, I made the decision to have something deeply meaningful to me inscribed on my right forearm. My family was initially quite dismayed when I told them. I think it shocked them more than anything. Regardless, their disapproval really rocked me. I had been so excited, and felt so empowered by this bold decision. It hurt that people I loved so much were not on board, bringing me to do some painful questioning of myself. I felt the need to capture their approval, to win them over to my side. While I can see why I did this (they eventually came around when they realized the full extent of what my tattoo meant to me), the problem was that this need to offer up an explanation didn't stop there.

For the longest time, I felt the need to capture the approval of every single person who asked about my tattoo. When I sensed disapproval, a feeling of discomfort would wash over me. I allowed their opinion of my tattoo to negatively impact my own opinion of my tattoo. As I've grown even more attached to and proud of it, I've come to discover the secret that *the more you love your decisions, the less you need others to love them.* Furthermore, *you are not required to validate your decisions or feelings to every person who asks about them.*

Now when random people ask me about my tattoo in passing, I tend to say something vague like, "It means I'm deep and edgy," give them a joking smile, and move forward. If they want to know more, sometimes I'll tell them more. But sometimes I don't, and when I don't, I feel comfortable with that decision.

We must stop believing that power and well-being are entities that come from outside ourselves, that our self-esteem and confidence depend on our being obedient to and measuring up to society's superficial requirements of us. We cannot let our inclinations toward the Effortless Perfection Myth steal our agency by convincing us that a life of pleasing, performing, and perfecting is the route to ultimate fulfillment when nothing could be farther from the truth.

When we look outside ourselves for validation, "the only change is an exchange of masters," notes Gloria Steinem. But when we look inside ourselves, "there is no need of masters."[8] We can stop grasping for the approval of an empty "Them." Instead of looking outward, we should be looking inward.

Section IV

Taking Up Space

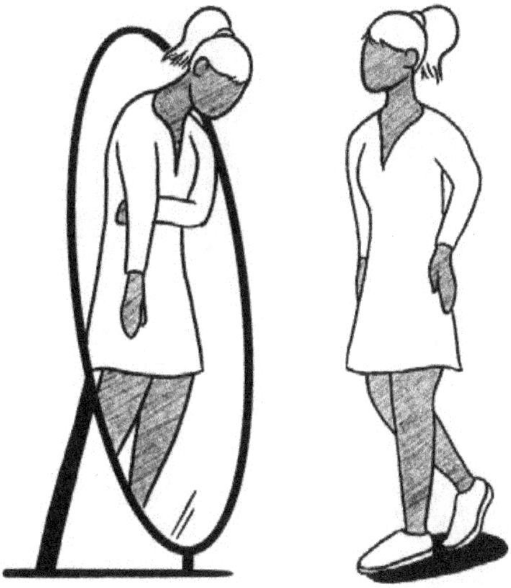

Chapter 20

Must Be This Thin to Ride

HAVE YOU EVER STARED AT A WORD for so long that it starts to look more like a jumbled mess of nonsensical letters, like something is wrong with it? I think women do something similar with their bodies when they stand in front of the mirror.

To say the typical female's relationship with her body is "complicated" would be an understatement. As women, we are taught from a young age that there is a great deal of value to be found in our bodies, but the extent of that value often depends on meeting oppressive standards dictated by outside forces. Not only does society impose strong opinions about what we should and should not be doing with our bodies, but it also places a heavy emphasis on how our bodies should and should not look. Which is why, even on high-achieving college campuses filled with young women who have the potential to change the world, many of us can also be found counting calories, obsessively high-tailing it to the gym, fat-shaming ourselves in mirrors, and generally going to war with our own bodies.

On some level, we all know that the behaviors we are engaging in are not exactly "healthy," per say. We know we are likely more obsessive and restrictive than we ought to be. But as we look around at all our peers em*body*ing Effortless Perfection with their flawless figures, we can't help but feel that we don't have a choice.

During my college experience, it wasn't exactly hard to miss that the first requirement of appearing Effortlessly Perfect was to be skinny. I felt like I'd shown up to an amusement park where instead of a sign reading "Must be this tall to ride," it said, "Must be this thin." I felt that if I didn't hit that marker, I wasn't getting on the ride. I believed my only other option would be to stare longingly from afar as my peers enjoyed the thrill.

Who could blame me and so many others for our willingness to push past the warning signs in our eagerness to make the cut? To sign the waiver without reading the fine print, throw our valuables in a locker, and get in line? We couldn't possibly allow ourselves to miss out on something that looks so fun!

But that's just the thing. What we don't know at the time is that *looks* fun doesn't necessarily always *feel* fun. Yeah, it *looks* fun to resemble Kate Moss, but the process it takes to get there and maintain that—of *feeling* that this needs to be our number-one priority—that's the true roller coaster. Sure, there will be exhilarating moments. That one picture at the bottom of the final drop will look amazing posted on social media! But there will also be numerous moments in which we feel nauseous and anxious, questioning why we ever chose to get strapped into this at all.

Still, we don't exactly feel able to voice our doubts to others. The moment we chose to get on board with Effortless Perfection was the moment we agreed to follow the unspoken rule about the struggles of maintaining a flawless exterior: If we don't bring up what's happening beneath the surface, nobody else will either. The Myth simply leaves no room for personal struggle or concern. Effortless Perfection is first and foremost about fitting an image, after all, and external appearance is the most integral part of that image. Thus, looking like we have it all is basically the same thing as actually having it all, right?

Wrong! Wrong! that little voice in the back of our head cries out. *That's not what you really believe, is it? You have so much more to offer the world than a skinny body. Where's your head?!* Suddenly, we are scolding ourselves for wanting something we've always told ourselves was superficial and for wanting it this badly. *We know better,* we tell ourselves. *This is not what we came to college to do or be. We came here to learn and grow and develop into young adults of whom we can be proud.* At least that's why we thought we were here.

Yet we still can't help but grow increasingly infuriated with ourselves for not being able to pull off that Effortlessly Perfect image. For not having the strength, or the willpower, or the self-discipline, or whatever it is we've convinced ourselves we are lacking, to achieve that figure we so strongly and inaccurately associate with the highest levels of success. We know we never should have allowed ourselves to believe it was something we could hold onto even if we could catch it. But... it's just really, really hard to let go.

Instead of letting go, the situation often progressively worsens as we are dragged further and further down the rabbit hole. According to a college-specific report released by the National Eating Disorders Association in 2013:

- Of the college women surveyed, 91 percent had attempted to control their weight through dieting,[1] with 82 percent engaging in one or more dieting behaviors on a daily basis.[2]
- Among "normal" dieters, 35 percent progressed to "pathological dieting."[3]
- Of those pathological dieters, 20–25 percent progressed to partial or full-symptom eating disorders.[4]

These numbers in calculation suggest that 8 percent of all female undergrads struggle with a diagnosable form of disordered eating. Most studies suggest half of those—so around 4 percent of all undergrad women—are full symptom.[5]

Notably, that percentage in relation to the total student population at a school usually rises as the institution's selectivity increases. Researchers and psychologists have confirmed that it is the young women considered high achievers who are the most likely to develop an eating disorder. A 2004 study on disordered eating at UPenn found that 60 percent of female students were trying to lose weight even though they were already at a healthy weight. Eating disorders there reportedly increased fourfold from 2001 to 2007. At Georgetown, as many as 25 percent of female students are thought to suffer from eating disorders. Duke is also no exception to such trends, with female students being found twice as likely to be diagnosed or treated for anorexia than the typical female college student.[6]

Effortless Perfection demands a self-discipline that acts as both the backbone of our successes in how it pushes us to always reach higher, as well as the bane of our existence in how it makes us so incredibly critical of ourselves, always pushing for better and never allowing us to be fully satisfied.

We don't recognize the slippery slope of behaviors that lead to an eating disorder because they are all so common that they look normal to us. Perhaps that's why only one in ten of those who suffer from an eating disorder receives treatment.[7] We have been taught to recognize only the extremes—the anorexic living on under 500 calories a day, the bulimic searching for a single stall bathroom in which to regurgitate lunch. But what about the majority of us who exist in a space that's not so straightforward? What about those of us who aren't stick-thin, who don't embody any of the stereotyped characteristics, but struggle nonetheless?

Disordered eating so often gets looked at as a black-and-white issue—either you have one or you don't, either you desperately need professional help or it's smooth sailing—when nothing could be further from the truth. Those of us who have been diagnosed with anorexia, bulimia, or another variation of disordered eating are not in some special category. We are merely individuals who are or were more extreme in our response to the constant pressures of a culture that emphasizes thinness and unobtainable beauty standards over individuality and health.

Courtney Martin writes in her book *Perfect Girls, Starving Daughters,* "Eating disorders are more [acute] versions of what nearly every girl and woman faces on a daily basis—a preoccupation with what they put in their mouths and how it affects the shape and size of their bodies."[8] Studies have found that up to 70 percent of college women report engaging in unhealthy behaviors, by utilizing extreme weight control techniques, including "chronic dieting, fasting, diuretics, or purging after eating."[9] These behaviors are not only common, they are routine.

To give a more specific example, 33 percent of college women report having employed serious weight control techniques such as vomiting or laxative use at least once a month.[10] Though these young women may not meet all the diagnostics for a full-blown disorder, they are still struggling with and suffering from many of the symptoms associated with disordered eating, such as "intense fear of gaining weight… feelings of ineffectiveness, a need to control one's environment, perfectionism, inflexible thinking, and restrained emotionality."[11] Their battle with body image is still dramatically impacting their quality of life in an immensely negative way.

The current way we perceive disordered eating—that it's not a problem until it suddenly is—needs to evolve. Struggles with body image and disordered eating would be much better understood if thought of as belonging to a continuum. Though official medical models appear to be moving in that direction, the way society perceives the issue is not.

It is critical that we do, because one does not have to be at the level of an eating disorder diagnosis to be powerfully affected. In a survey by Clover Letter, an online newsletter for girls ages fifteen to twenty-two, almost 40 percent of respondents reported they were distracted by thoughts of thier own appearance at least six times a day, and one in five admitted being distracted ten times or more a day.[12]

"How I feel about my body on a given day bleeds itself into my experience; maybe positive, maybe negative, but it's way too much either way," notes Jordan. Her awareness of and concern about her body is a cognitive burden that follows her around like a cloud—a negative voice relentlessly at the ready to berate her. To great detriment, she has internalized the sense that the shape of her body plays a vital role in determining her value.

This desire for value, and the lengths we are willing to go for it, only increases as we watch those around us dedicate themselves to taking on this burden as well, having deemed it a worthy cause. Melissa remarks, "My senior year, my best friend had an eating disorder and then that summer I went to visit my cousin and she was the same way, and it made me feel like maybe I should have an eating disorder. I was noticing their habits and how they were losing weight, and as a teenage girl I just thought, okay, that's what we are all doing and supposed to be doing."

Notice the way Melissa's recollection paints such an unhealthy state of mind as something to aspire to, rather than something from which to protect oneself. This is a major red flag about the way society views the issue—particularly impressionable young women! Disordered eating is not an advantageous triumph; it is a disease that can kill you.

Even those who understand this key fact often find themselves struggling. Katie has seen with her own eyes the havoc that eating disorders can wreak, having grown up "surrounded" by people who had unhealthy relationships with their bodies. She places a high priority on maintaining a healthy mindset. Though she tries her best not to engage in any behaviors associated with disordered eating, she still has not been able to outwit the body dysmorphia that typically tags along with the disease. (Body dysmorphia is a clinical term describing the inability to stop thinking about a body flaw that is either minor or imagined.)[13]

She confesses, "Day to day, the number of girls I stare at—like, 'I wish I could be you,' 'wish I could have that body part like your legs or abs'—is staggering." She's happy with how she looks "in theory," but there are certain areas she sometimes finds herself repetitively taking stock of, judging how they "stick out" in ways she does not find satisfactory. Katie has a hard time seeing her body the way everyone else sees it, which is a desirably curvy and able body. Her eyes are drawn to her flaws.

In the same way the Effortless Perfection Myth blinds us from reality and sets us up to see ourselves as failures, body dysmorphia and disordered eating push us into a constant state of unfounded insecurity. We are kept on edge about where we stand, feeling like we must remain constantly vigilant over our bodies, lest we lose any hard-won ground. There's never a moment to lay our weapons down and stop fighting.

If I were to pinpoint the one feeling central to an eating disorder, I'd say it is *distrust*. A distrust in our own bodies not to betray us by taking a new shape outside the one we feel is societally demanded of us. A distrust of what the world will do to us, how it will treat us, if we do not embody perfection and respectability in its eyes. Because of this, our bodies come to feel like cages we are captured inside, as opposed to manifestations of our very being through which we get to experience the world.

We cannot let such a mindset go unchallenged. We must continuously remind ourselves that all the time and energy we spend worrying about our weight and our appearance, the disappointment that infiltrates our emotional being every time we disapprovingly evaluate ourselves in the mirror—all that mars our ability to maintain healthy self-esteem, confidence, and self-love. And we need all of these to lead productive, fulfilling, empowered lives.

To push back against the Effortless Perfection Myth, we need to get out of our heads and back into our bodies. By rekindling our relationship with our material senses and listening to our bodily urges, we reject the following tenets of the Myth: *Perfectionism has no room for human hungers. You must tame your desires out of you. Anything that introduces the potential for unruliness must go. You must will your way to perfection by striking back against any part of you that threatens to pull you off the path. You must show your dedication to perfection by denying and detesting that which does not feed the ultimate goal of appearing outwardly flawless.*

It's time to call BS.

So how do we show Effortless Perfection that we aren't having any of it? We reenter our bodies by daring ourselves to feel all the things it is trying to tell us: *I'm hurt, I'm hungry, I'm more than Enough.* We recognize the extent to which our ability to participate in the world around us has been fettered by discomfort with, and perhaps even outright hatred of, our own bodily vessels. We allow ourselves time to mourn what we've lost in our quest for Effortless Perfection and then we make a promise to ourselves that it will claim no more!

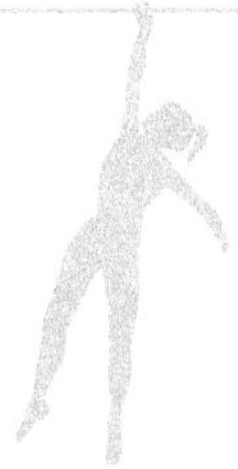

Chapter 21

Anorexia Is Not the Only Eating Disorder

THE LONG-HELD ASSUMPTION that you can "tell" when someone has an eating disorder by looking at them is simply not true. Disordered eating is just as much about what is going on inside one's mind as it is about how one's body appears on the outside. Subsequently, another assumption that needs to evolve is the belief that disordered eating only comes in one form—anorexia, which involves excessive food restriction. On the contrary, multiple other forms exist:

- *Bulimia* involves bingeing (consuming excessive amounts of food) and purging (via vomiting, taking laxatives, or over-exercising).
- *Binge eating disorder* involves feeling a loss of control around food, often resulting in consuming unusually large amounts of food in a short period of time. (Though those who struggle with this variation of disordered eating don't purge afterward, they often feel deep shame or guilt about the behavior.)
- *Orthorexia* involves an unhealthy obsession with healthy or "clean" eating.
- *Pica* involves craving and chewing non-food substances with no nutritional value like ice, clay, soil, or paper.
- *Eating disorder not otherwise specified (EDNOS)* involves a

combination of symptoms from the aforementioned eating disorders, but may not meet exact criteria.

It's important to recognize the wide range of eating disorders that exist (the scope of which expands beyond those discussed above). Each are equally valid. Each come with unique struggles worth recognizing and addressing; not doing so often leaves those in need of care to fend for themselves.

For instance, a friend of mine who struggled with bingeing and purging felt incredibly invalidated upon taking the courageous step to open up and tell her father she had an eating disorder, only to be told, "I watched you eat a whole candy bar yesterday, so I find that hard to believe." In responding this way, he rejected her call for help—and made her wary of asking for help in the future—because her form of disordered eating did not meet stereotypical behaviors (i.e. it did not look like anorexia). He misunderstood that there is more than one way of expressing upheaval occurring within one's mind and body.

Binge eating disorder is another form of disordered eating that comes with unique hardships. Lily at Duke has battled with binge eating disorder from a young age, leading to weight gain that has placed her struggle very visibly on the outside of her and has drawn a great deal of unwanted attention. In a piece entitled "#Exile," she writes that she has learned to cope with things like the "cold glares" on a full-to- capacity bus where "no one wants to sit next to me because one of my thighs is taking up the entire seat" and the "snickering behind me when I wear leggings" by seeking refuge in her phone and laptop everywhere she goes. Constantly bracing for rejection, she notes, "If I keep my face down and my ears plugged, I won't see the disdain in people's eyes when they are flabbergasted by how much excess weight I am carrying."

Painfully aware of the very obvious standard of beauty at Duke, a standard Lily in no way feels she fits into, the most infuriating thing for her is witnessing those who *do* fit into that standard complain about a "small roll on their stomach" or a "little bat wing on their arms." Countless times she has watched as girls have publicly announced to their friends while riding on the campus bus or inspecting themselves in a public restroom mirror, "Oh my God—I'm getting so fat! I need to hit the gym immediately before I become obese." Every time this occurs it makes Lily feel like screaming:

> *NEWSFLASH, BITCH! You're not fat! You are not fat! You are the size of a toothpick. Just because you have a wrinkle on your stomach, you want to complain?! I WILL GIVE YOU SOMETHING TO COMPLAIN ABOUT! You wanna know what fat is? Fat is exile! It is banishment. It is everyone, and I mean everyone, not even giving you a chance to just be. It is being stuck between the most invasive and constant examination and consigned to the darkest invisibility. It is the assumption you don't care, and because you don't care, you're not worth me caring about you.*

Lily is often frustrated by how blissfully unaware so many are of what it actually feels like to be obese. Especially when nothing she does ever feels truly "acceptable."

If she orders a salad, she gets giggles. If she orders the chicken quesadilla with extra cheese, she's made fun of. Every time she walks into the gym, she can feel that stares of the "normal-bodied" following her from machine to machine. And all she wants to do is turn around and scream: "I'm doing the best I can!" Her primary struggle is about far more than her body; it is about being denied the feeling of worthiness by others because of her body. And, as Lindy West writes in her book *Shrill*, "Denying people access to value is an incredibly insidious form of emotional violence."[1]

The judgment of others regarding her size has cut Lily deeply on too many occasions to count. On one such occasion, she was sitting in a lecture-room discussion for an ethics class of over a hundred people when a fellow student voiced a strong opinion that essentially boiled down to "when I see fat people, I see laziness." Lily expounds:

> *It may not have been his exact wording, but it was like he was saying that people like me were not worthy of general human respect, or at least that's how I left the room feeling. I was fuming mad. I had dealt with people's opinions and judgments about how I look in elementary school, middle school, high school, and now here I was at a college I had busted my ass to get into and people were still drawing unfair conclusions.*

How did earning a spot at a top-ten school not nullify any and all beliefs that she wasn't a dedicated and incredibly hard worker? And what did this guy know about her personal exercise regimen and the other extensive efforts she made to be healthy?

Her frustration here is beyond valid. Authors such as Lindy West and Roxane Gay have written in great depth about the pain of having their extra weight so often regarded by others as both an intellectual and even a moral failure. Lily's comments confirm this: "There's the laziness component of judgment from others, like I already said, but there's also the beauty component where we make judgments about how smart and nice people probably are based off of their appearance." Thus, she concludes, beauty is both a privilege and a commodity in our society. It's a form of social capital that gets read into far further than it deserves, especially where the expectations and pressures of Effortless Perfection are concerned.

Lily is certainly not alone in this belief. All the women I interviewed who struggled with their weight had the same criticism that "it's almost as though, until your vessel 'passes,' nothing else about you matters." The way our society makes those in this position feel is simply unacceptable.

Furthermore, Lily points out how, even when we *do* bring up issues of disordered eating and Effortless Perfection on campus, it is "always through the lens of a white girl struggling with bulimia and anorexia, and there's nothing wrong with having that narrative, but there are other ones, too." Representation matters. Lily's story is an important counter-narrative to the traditional notion of what disordered eating looks like.

She demonstrates how "when the lights are turned on, we all have something we are struggling with" and just because she binge-eats and the other girl vomits after she eats, does not mean they are not "on flip sides of the same coin." Lily insists that the best way to start the healing process is to "come out of the proverbial closet about what we are feeling and experiencing, and hear this multiplicity of stories and let them give us freedom."

It is time we stop viewing disordered eating as some unremarkable rite of passage. There is nothing normal about feeling this level of hatred toward one's own body. We cannot let Effortless Perfection convince us otherwise.

Chapter 22

The Big Bad Media

MY THERAPIST ONCE TOLD ME, "You aren't the one with an eating disorder. Society has an eating disorder. You are just suffering from the side effects." He could not have been more right. Looking around at the intense emphasis women's appearance receives, day in and day out, it is understandable that we all struggle in our own ways to maintain healthy perspective in a world that likes to constantly remind us that our bodies are far from Effortlessly Perfect.

We are *constantly* being barraged with messages conveying the notion that a woman's value lies in her body and her ability to mold it to fit the "ideal" feminine form. For instance, in the top 500 films from 2007 to 2012, only 30.8 percent of speaking characters were women, and roughly a third of those speaking characters were shown in "sexually revealing attire" or at least "partially naked." Also, 28.8 percent of all the female actors in these top 500 films wore sexually revealing clothes, as opposed to 7 percent of male actors, and 26.2 percent of female actors got at least partially naked as opposed to 9.4 percent of male actors.[1] In media, all too often our role as women is to act as nothing more than hypersexualized bodies—ornamental commodities, prizes to be won, even possessions to be conquered. We are to be seen, but not heard.

Watching female bodies being displayed in this way is believed to have a direct correlation with body image issues. Dr. Anne Becker was the first to demonstrate this in her 1995–1998 Fiji study, which surveyed secondary school girls on the island as Western television—think *Baywatch, Melrose Place,* and *Beverly Hills 90210*—first made its way to their region of the globe.

Before 1995, the year satellites began beaming television signals over, there was little talk of dieting in Fiji. "The idea of calories was very foreign to them," Erica Goode writes in a *New York Times* article on the study.[2] But over the course of three years, rates of disordered eating behaviors on the island skyrocketed. By 1998, 69 percent of women surveyed said that at some time they had been on a diet.

Goode further details, "15 percent in the 1998 survey reported that they had induced vomiting to control their weight…compared with 3 percent in the 1995 survey. And 29 percent scored highly on a test of eating-disorder risk, compared with 13 percent just three years before."[3] What's more, "[g]irls who said they watched television three or more nights a week in the 1998 survey were 50 percent more likely to describe themselves as 'too big or fat' and 30 percent more likely to diet than girls who watched television less frequently."[4]

Clearly these images of excessively skinny women have a measurable effect on those consuming the images. We can't call them harmless. They are a form of subliminal messaging enforcing the Effortless Perfection Myth. They plant unrealistic ideas in our head about what's attractive and what we are meant to aspire to.

Don't even get me started about the messaging in music videos, which are constantly reinforcing the notion that women are objects rather than whole human beings. Since their widespread broadcast began (MTV aired in 1981), "music videos—like other forms of advertising—have relied heavily on stories concerning female sexuality to fulfill their function of selling CDs and albums for record companies," explains Sut Jhally in the documentary *Dream Worlds 3*.[5] Frames focus on just our asses, our legs, our boobs, our lips—effectively dismembering our bodies down into parts detached from the wholeness of the entity to which they belong. The final product tends to look awfully similar to the way women are presented in pornography. (Porn stars even have a history of starring in music videos!)[6]

Beyond the film and music industries, the messages dispersed to women by print advertisements, billboards, and television commercials about the utter importance of possessing hot, sexualized bodies are inescapable. The constant bombardment of Photoshopped, airbrushed images reminding us of how we are "meant" to look is relentless.

It's quite honestly the widest-reaching public service announcement ever to have existed. We can no longer turn a corner at the mall or on a big city street without seeing an objectifying ad of a woman being "used to sell something (anything)—and really what's being sold is her."[7] This problem is so rampant that we've stopped even giving it a second thought, but that doesn't mean it has ceased having an impact on the way we see ourselves and our place in a culture that is so nonchalant about the objectification of women.

These images are testaments to the extent to which the female body and female sexuality are shamelessly exploited to draw attention to and sell products:

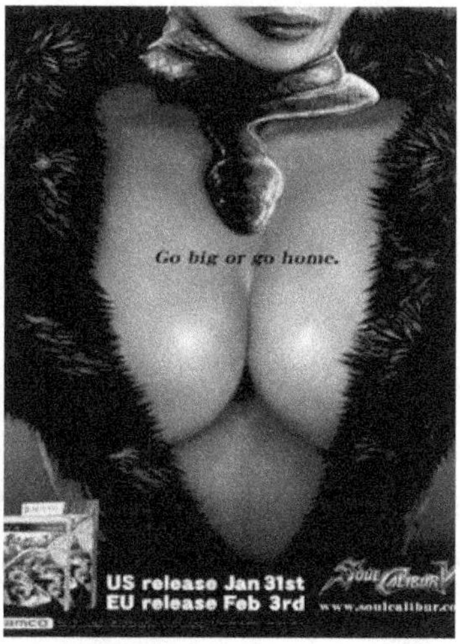

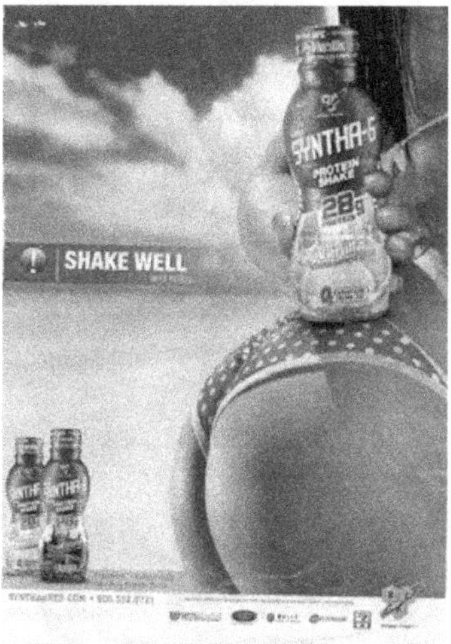

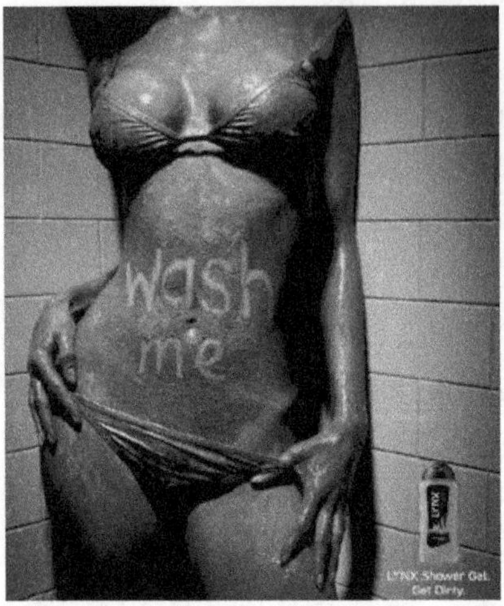
wash me
LYNX Shower Gel.
Get Dirty.

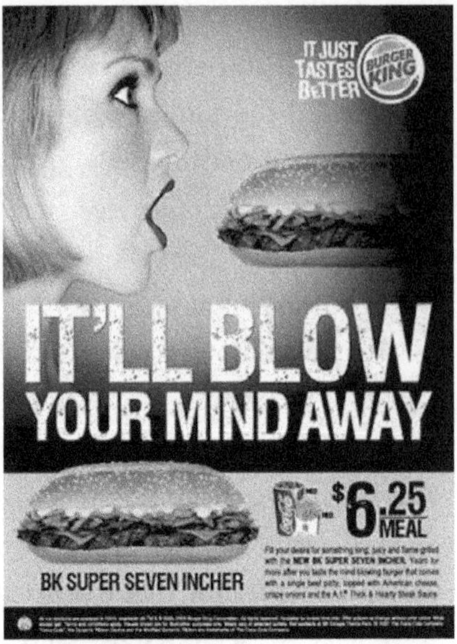
IT JUST TASTES BETTER
BURGER KING
IT'LL BLOW YOUR MIND AWAY
$6.25 MEAL
BK SUPER SEVEN INCHER

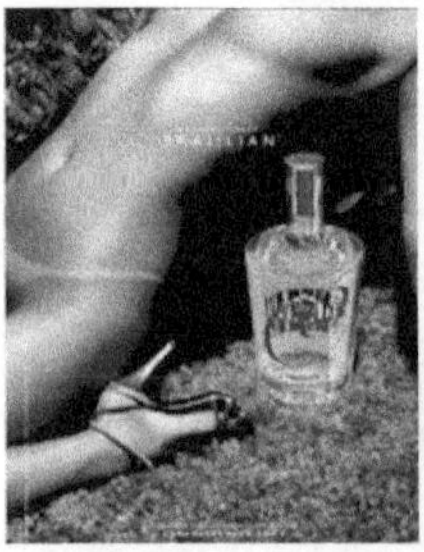

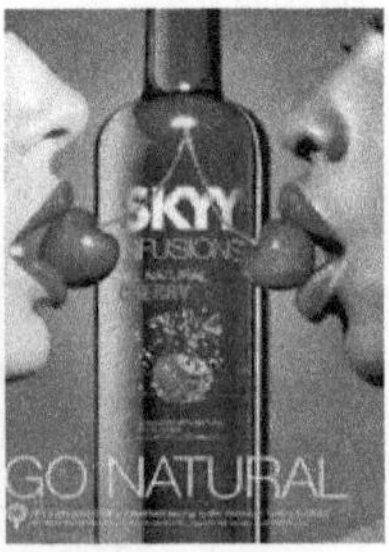
SKYY
INFUSIONS
GO NATURAL

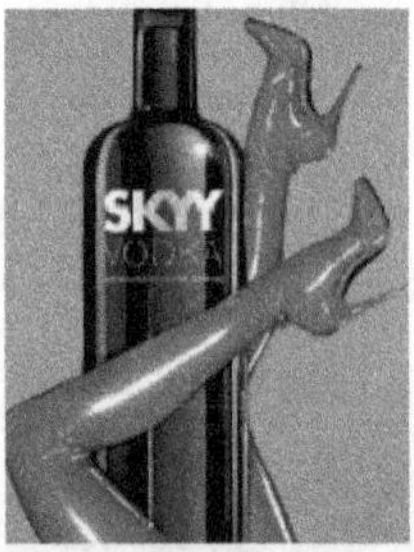
SKYY
VODKA

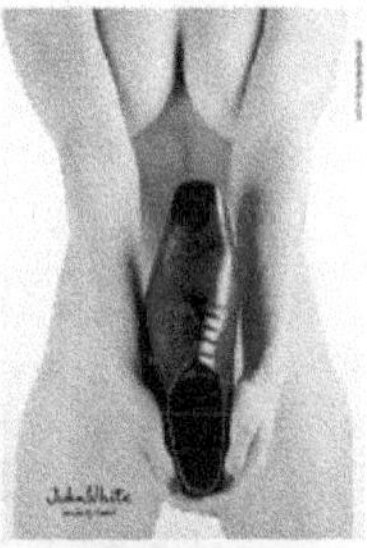

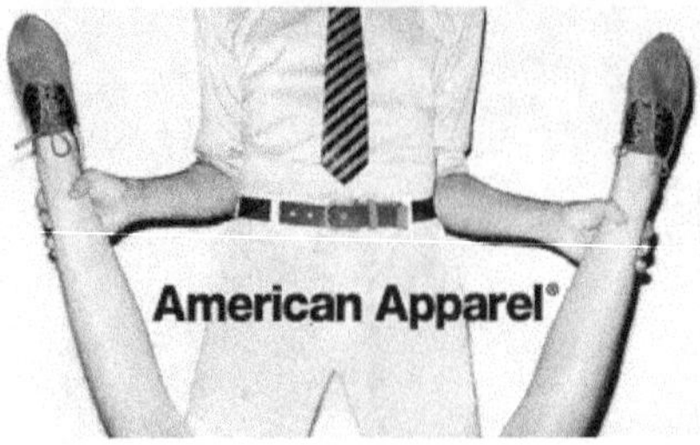
American Apparel®

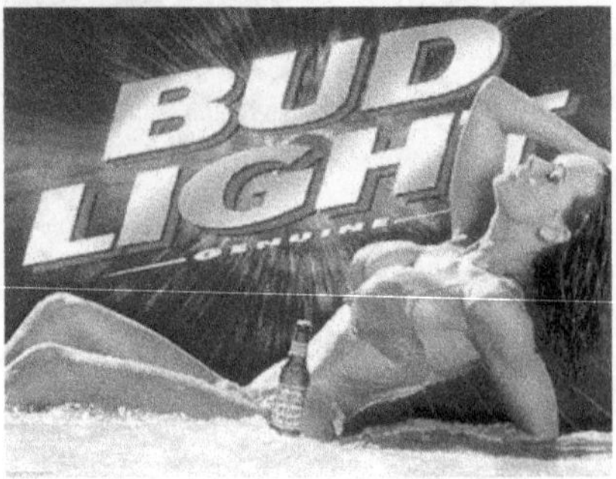
BUD LIGHT
GENUINE

Upon asking the young women I interviewed how these images made them feel, the responses were unsurprisingly all negative. Abby remarked, "If I could talk to the people who made all these ads I'd ask them, 'If you had a daughter, what do you think she would think when looking at this? Is this the type of value you want to instill in your child? Because that's what you are basically instilling in all of society by putting this out there.'"

Francesca's analysis of the images used in these advertisements was also powerful and thought-provoking:

> *These are all pretty gross. The one about the seven-inch sandwich that will "blow your mind away"—that does not in any way make me want to eat that sandwich. Hello! Women buy these products too. At least try to make your ads palatable for us. And the ones for Skyy vodka are so...well...phallic! I don't want to imagine my vodka as a penis. Does anyone? But the concept behind having a women's legs wrapped around the bottle in that way or placing the two girls' mouths right there is definitely supposed to invoke that.*

Her point is alarmingly accurate. When considering the way both genders tend to be postured and positioned in ads, these images clearly reinforce the particularly demeaning narrative that women's bodies are meant for passive display while men's bodies should be used for action.

Francesca's media literacy[i] calls out the strong "ick factor" behind these ads' motifs. And yet, if you think those are bad, try Googling

[i] Media literacy—or the ability to analyze and assess media, particularly the harmful biases and misrepresentations it often depicts—is crucial to protecting our mental health and sense of what is real. I recommend watching the documentaries *Miss Representation*, *Killing Us Softly*, and *Dream Worlds 3*, as well as looking at online resources like IREX's "Learn to Discern" media literacy training program and the News Literacy Project's Checkology program for more information.

"objectifying ads" and taking a gander at what pops up. Tom Ford, Alexander Wang, American Apparel, Dolce & Gabbana, Fresh One, RedTape, and Lynx are some of the worst offenders. Beer, hard liquor, and car advertisements can be pretty appalling, as well.

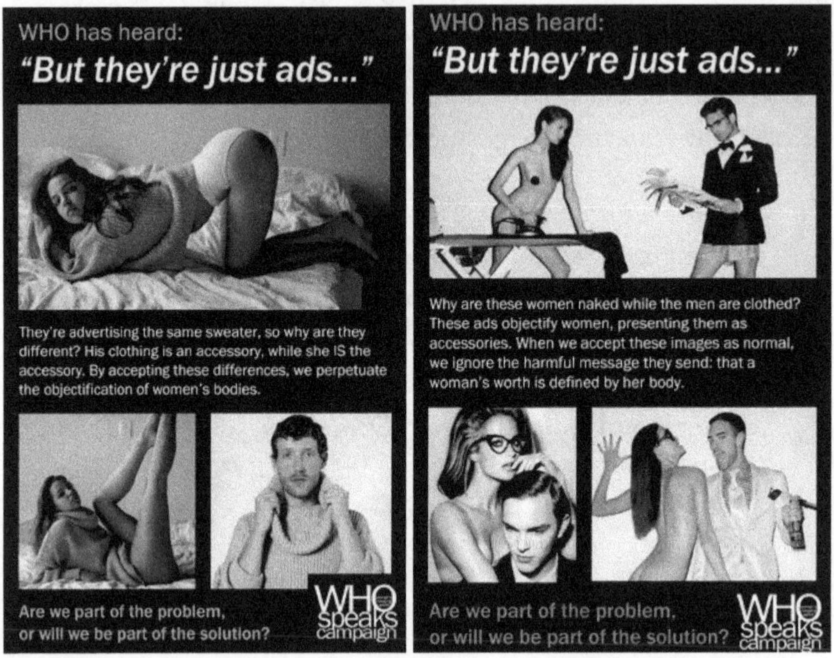

In 2014, a student group at Duke known as the Women's Housing Option (WHO) put together a campus-wide poster campaign called "WHO Speaks" to bring attention to the extent that advertisements objectify female bodies. WHO notes that picturing men fully clothed and women largely naked in the same image demonstrates that "his clothing is an accessory, while she *is the accessory."*

When female bodies aren't being used to sell products to men via sexual allurement, they are being used to sell products to women by intentionally making us self-conscious about our skin, hair, figures, you name it, and preying on those insecurities in an attempt to make us bigger consumers.

First consider that U.S. ad expenditure was $240.7 billion in 2019.[8] Then consider that an overwhelming percentage of advertising campaigns feature female models who, on average, already weigh 23 percent less than the standard American woman[9] and are then Photoshopped to look even thinner, more toned, and more glamorous. Advertisers want to create the illusion that this kind of Effortlessly Perfect appearance is "the norm," that women are meant to look like this and anything less is reason for rejection.

A huge part of the advertising business depends on making us feel unattractive. *I repeat: a major corporate strategy is to make us feel unattractive; it's called "insecure consumerism."* Advertisers intentionally make the standard of beauty as narrow as possible because, if that standard were to "acknowledge a variety of beauties," then women would spend far less money on beauty products, diet books, miracle pills, spandex, and the like.[10] An article entitled "Commodity Feminism" in a well-known academic journal notes that, though the strategies of commercialization have changed over time, ads targeted at women are still designed to create "idealized definitions of feminine desirability that [are] always just beyond reach" to play on women's self-esteem.[11]

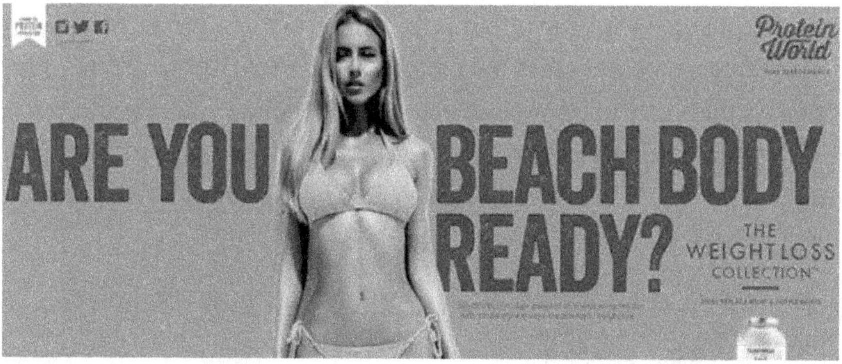

Looks to me like a super-effective way to make women self-conscious of their bodies!

In regard to weight and body image, this "out-of-reach" component of corporate strategy has, in part, been implemented through the promotion of a body type that is at least ten to fifteen pounds below the point where women's bodies are naturally set to be, and then redefining our natural womanly shapes as "too fat." Thus, many of us are kept in constant battle with bodies that are just struggling to maintain a healthy BMI, giving advertisers the perfect hook to sell their products by promising a solution to all our woes—woes that they intentionally cultivated in the first place.

If this sounds too much like a "conspiracy theory" for you, consider that when *The Feminine Mystique* came out and the second wave of the feminist movement was launched, much of what women's magazines had traditionally held to be their area of expertise (housekeeping, childrearing, cooking) was suddenly deemed less relevant. They needed to find a new way to sell magazines, and fast.

In her book *The Beauty Myth*, Naomi Wolf writes, "In a stunning move, an entire replacement culture was developed by naming a 'problem' where it had scarcely existed before."[12] As a result, the number of diet-related articles in magazines skyrocketed over this time period; from 1968 to 1972, they rose a stunning 70 percent. "'The lucrative transfer of guilt' was resurrected just in time," Wolf asserts. "Somehow, somewhere, someone must have figured out that [women] buy more things if they are kept in the self-hating, ever-failing, hungry, and sexually insecure state of being aspiring 'beauties.'"[13] Since then, things have only gotten worse. The increasingly stringent expectations enforced by the Effortless Perfection Myth certainly have not helped.

Whenever I find myself feeling badly about my body, I ask myself, *Who does this feeling benefit? Is it some corporation trying to profit off my body insecurities?* If so, *what would I say to the CEO of that company if he were saying to my face what I am currently thinking to myself?* If he were to approach me in his gray suit and slicked back hair and say, "You're too fat for those jeans" or "You don't have the bust for that dress", *how would I respond?* I'd likely have some expletives to share with him. So, why not take that anger at that fictional (or not so fictional) character and tell the negative social forces inside my head making me feel so badly about my body to scram?

The beauty, dieting, and advertising industries are not all that interested in women as leaders and changemakers. They are only interested in women as consumers and will do everything it takes to make us consume, even if that means *intentionally* undermining our body confidence. This lack of confidence, unfortunately, tends to bleed into all other aspects of our lives.

Research has shown that concerns with weight and body image, as they grow in intensity, almost always lead to "a virtual collapse of self-esteem and sense of effectiveness."[14] The fact that thirty-three thousand American women reported that they would rather lose ten to fifteen pounds than achieve any other goal is incredibly distressing.[15] Also disturbing is the finding that "over ½ the females between the ages of 18–25 would prefer to be run over by a truck than be fat, and ⅔ surveyed would rather be mean or stupid."[16] Could our priorities possibly be any more warped?

This is all ludicrous! And it is no doubt linked to the manner in which we are constantly being force-fed the notion that our power lies in our youth, beauty, and sexuality, *rather than our capacity to be good people and make positive, effective contributions to the world.*

What's worse, when we do see women who are making strides as leaders and political movers-and-shakers, the media feels it necessary to belittle them through the use of sexualizing commentary that no man in a similar position has ever had to face to the same extreme, if at all.

The media does things like ask prominent female politicians on live television if they've had breast implants (2008 vice-presidential candi-date Sarah Palin), make comments like "I think even if you waterboarded [her], she wouldn't admit to plastic surgery" (Speaker of the House Nancy Pelosi), hypersexualize their fashion choices by commenting on the exposure of a half-inch of breast line (2016 presidential candidate Hillary Clinton), or call them a dominatrix for wearing knee-high black boots to work one day (former Secretary of Defense Condoleezza Rice).

The documentary Miss Representation begs the question, "The fact that media are so limiting and so derogatory to the MOST powerful women in the country...what does it say about media's ability to take any woman in America seriously?"[17]

Being taken seriously should not be some cookie given to and taken away from us depending on whether we look good or bad, put together or haggard, sexy or asexual. This is a strategy that has been used time and time again to take attention off the issues that we as women are pushing, by minimizing us along with our arguments.

We need to redirect our energies from fighting to appear Effortlessly Perfect so that others will give us respect and instead fight the entities demanding that respectability be tied to the impossible standard of Effortless Perfection in the first place.

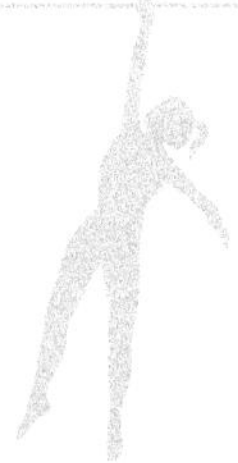

Chapter 23
Whose Body Is This, Anyway?

IN ADDITION TO THE WAY WE SEE the female form in general being treated and commented on (via popular culture and mainstream media), how we relate to our bodies is also heavily impacted by the way we personally experience *our own* female form being treated and commented on (via everyday happenings).

Our posture. Our complexion. Our wardrobe. Whether we count as attractive. What level of attractiveness we are (1–10). What size our boobs are. How round our asses are. Whether we're trying too hard. Whether we're not trying hard enough. How much we eat. How little we eat. How much weight we've gained. How much weight we've lost. We are under constant scrutiny for all of these things, often without us even being involved in the conversation, without having even uttered a word to provoke the discussion or being given a chance to defend ourselves.

Feminist author Scaachi Koul writes, "It's rarely you decide there's something wrong with you; instead, you get your cues from someone who is the right combination of bored, cruel, and insecure about themselves to begin with."[1] All it takes is overhearing something you weren't meant to hear to trigger the development of serious body insecurities. I have a vivid memory from high school of my boyfriend at the time excitedly picking me up and spinning me around in a circle after having not seen each other for a couple of days. In the midst of this cute display of affection, I was distracted by a loud outburst of laughter down the hall coming from a group of guys on my track team.

"What was so funny?" I asked one of them two minutes later on the way to class.

"Nothing, nothing," he said uneasily.

"Dude," I replied. "Tell me."

After an awkward silence, he mumbled, "One of the guys said he bet Dan wished he could squeeze all the fat off you." As if to suggest that was why my boyfriend had given me such an extravagant hug.

"Oh," I choked back. I was by no means overweight, but that clearly didn't matter. I was fair game for being made the subject of these kinds of hurtful remarks.

Comments such as these tend to start young. Multiple young women I interviewed could pinpoint the exact year they heard their first cutting remark. Many even remembered the setting and the name of the person who said it, while also admitting they could remember little else about that period of their lives with such clarity. Abby notes, "The first time was in sixth grade. It was around the time guys started rating girls on a hotness scale from one to ten. A popular girl asked a popular guy what I was and he said a four. Ben Sampson was his name…I'll never forget."

These two scenarios may seem like "little things" that were said a "long time ago," but they no doubt worked their way into the body concepts Abby and I had for ourselves as young women (and possibly even now).

In her book *Appetites: Why Women Want*, Caroline Knapp addresses the confusion girls face as we grow into our bodies and experience all the perplexing reactions and judgments that come along with that development:

> *The body—this mysterious, secretive, unpredictable thing that boys seemed to admire and respond to nonetheless—became a source of power and also a source of the most profound confusion... it could confirm value, but only a particular kind, one that needed to be managed—seized and sexualized—in order to be brought into existence. This is a fearsome combination; power is scary when you're not sure how deeply it runs, when you're not convinced it even exists beneath the thin waist and the shiny hair, when it needs to be constantly reinforced by other people, whose judgment you may not even trust.*[2]

Because we don't know what to make of our newly developed bodies as young women, we end up giving others the power to conclude an opinion for us. We grow to distrust our own vision, leading us to look to others to assure us that we are beautiful and desirable. Those dang reassurance addictions are at it again, stoking the flames of Effortless Perfection: *Am I good enough? How do I confirm my worth?*

WHO Speaks launched a second campaign in 2012 to demonstrate the constant commentary young women receive on our bodies and how it leads us to question ourselves and our place in the environments we inhabit.[3]

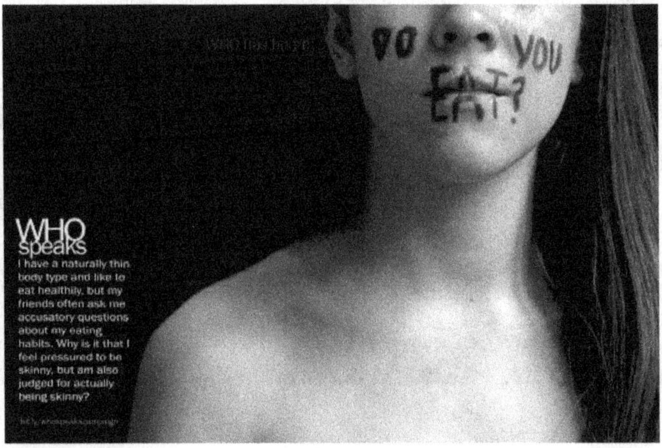

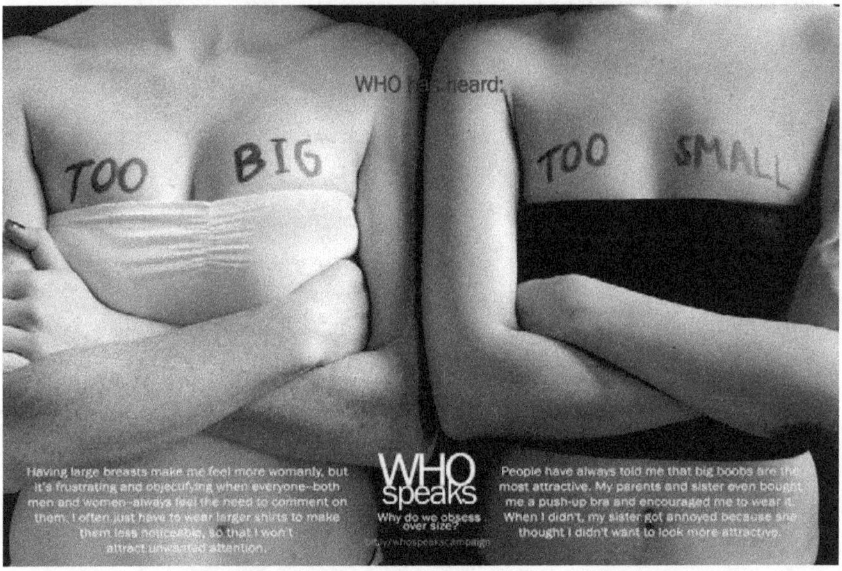
TOO BIG
TOO SMALL
Having large breasts make me feel more womanly, but it's frustrating and objecufying when everyone--both men and women--always feel the need to comment on them. I often just have to wear larger shirts to make them less noticeable, so that I won't attract unwanted attention.
WHO speaks
Why do we obsess over size?
People have always told me that big boobs are the most attractive. My parents and sister even bought me a push-up bra and encouraged me to wear it. When I didn't, my sister got annoyed because she thought I didn't want to look more attractive.

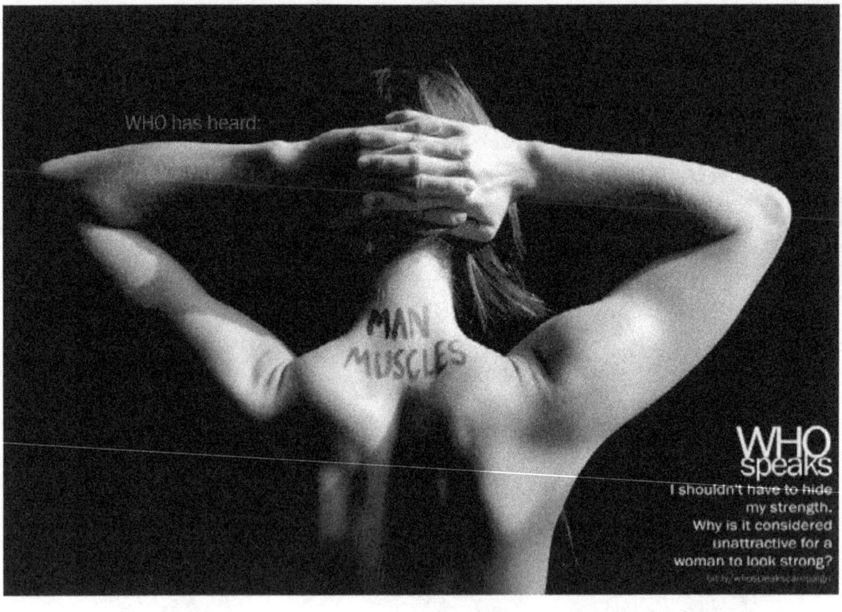
WHO has heard:
MAN MUSCLES
WHO speaks
I shouldn't have to hide my strength.
Why is it considered unattractive for a woman to look strong?

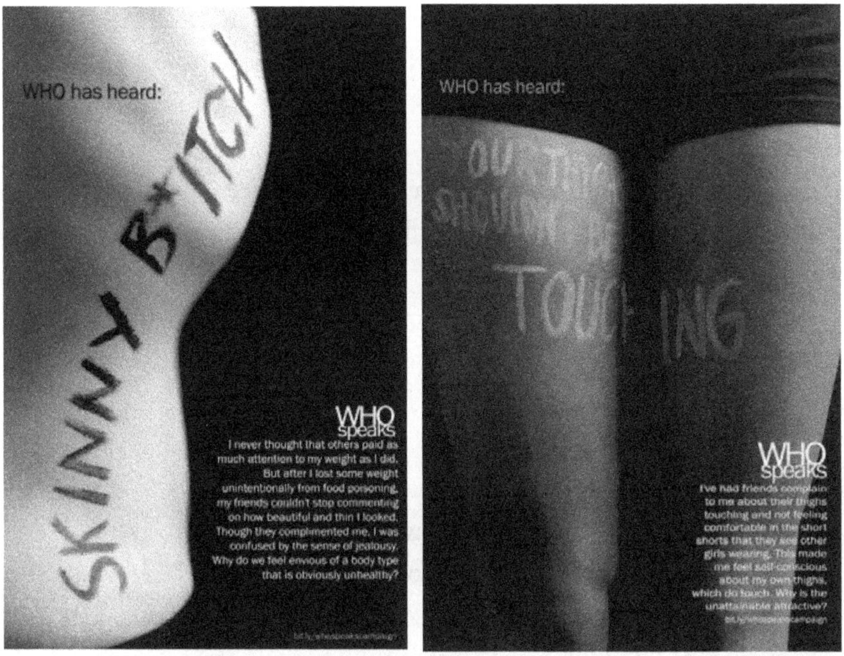

Residing within a female figure is no easy task. We live in a society that feels entitled to go out of its way to comment on female appearance, constantly. Unfortunately, this also includes how women speak to other women. For Katie, many damaging comments came from her mom and sister suggesting she go work out or remarking on how her clothes fit. "Maybe these were little things, but they definitely came from the people closest to me, which—if I think about it—is kinda fucked up," she reflects.

When it comes to our bodies, women have a really hard time relating to and interacting with one another. Discussions about body image with female peers all too often devolve into fat talk and harmful comparisons. Naomi Wolf reminds us that, while consumer culture promotes the myth that women must look flawlessly beautiful in order to be accepted, "it would be powerless if women didn't enforce [that myth] against one another."[4] And, if you really think about it, we are enforcing it on each other *all the time.*

We enforce it upon each other every time engage in the ritual language of self-hatred that is fat talk, as we habitually exchange self-inflicted insults about our legs, our stomachs, our arms, our chins for the sense of faux intimacy that comes from collectively beating ourselves up and pretending it makes us feel better. We enforce it upon ourselves when we excessively talk about how much we've eaten, how little we've exercised, how "good" or "bad" we've been on a given day.

In short, we enforce it upon each other when we allow it to become a main staple of everyday conversation. It's okay to want to talk about bodily insecurities, but we need to be aware of how often and in what ways we go about doing so. A 2011 study by Rachel Salk and Renee Engeln-Maddox revealed that 90 percent of female undergrads engage in fat talk, even though only 9 percent are overweight.[5] No wonder college women are the most at-risk group for developing eating disorders![6] Not to mention, habitual fat talk among friend groups is especially cruel to overweight girls in the circle, as Lily pointed out earlier in Chapter 21, because it is a constant reminder that other girls are scared of "being what I am…scared of being me."

Fat talk forces women into spaces of comparison and competition. Women cycle through an awkward, self-deprecating form of call-and-response:

"God, I wish I had your legs, mine are just so flabby."

"I don't know what you are talking about. I'd trade my boobs for yours any day."

"Oh whatever. My arms are what I hate the most. They have no tone."

"What? You are crazy! Look at how bad mine are!"

Each remark is met with an assurance to the person who expressed it, followed by a negation aimed at oneself. The objective here may feel like joint commiseration, but there's something deeper. Those involved are homing in on and breaking down every aspect of their bodies in incredibly unforgiving and judgmental ways.

Which is exactly what the Effortless Perfection Myth wants. The Myth wants to pit us against each other in a quest to feel good enough, fighting to qualify for the attention and praise this standardized beauty promises to bring. It wants us to see other women as possible aggressors, rather than allies. And nobody, not even the girl considered most beautiful, wins when this is the setup.

The real way we all win? We pay attention to the language we are using. We stop policing our own and each other's bodies. We give ourselves and other women permission to do the things we crave—to eat what we want, wear what we want, embrace our different body types—without constant commentary.

This is easiest when we've first learned to love our own bodies. We are much less likely to be manipulated into caring about the choices other women make in relation to how they dress, pose, or appear if we are content with our own choices. And with all the body-image crap that gets thrown at us from everywhere else, we can't afford not to be on the same team here.

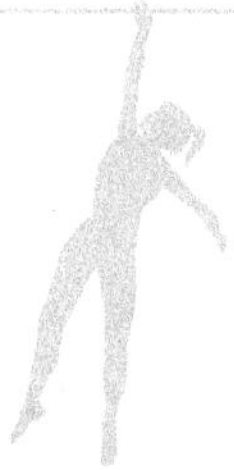

Chapter 24

Racialized Beauty Standards

SPEAKING OF CELEBRATING multiple different body types, it is critical to note the way in which our country's media reinforces a very narrow and *racialized* standard of beauty. For numerous reasons, we cannot discuss body image issues and disordered eating without discussing race.

First, there tend to be different body type ideals according to race, which can lead to different behavioral manifestations of disordered eating. As previously stated, you can't just look someone up and down and assume you know they are struggling with the disease. It comes in many forms.

Second, cultural factors may cause some racial groups to hold greater taboo against disordered eating due to its stereotype as a white women's disease; thus, women of color are less likely to accept or seek help when they need it. For instance, Black girls' body issues often do not draw the attention they deserve because they have "stereotypically been thought to be relatively immune to eating disorders and the thin ideal."[1] However, meta-analysis by Shelby Grabe and Janet Hyde of over a hundred studies revealed that woman of color struggle the same amount as white women. Hispanic and Asian American girls have actually been found to struggle with body image the most.[2]

Third, the Western world abides by a white standard of beauty. Don't believe me? Consider how women of color are severely underrepresented in U.S. media despite the fact that over a third of our country's population is not white.[3] Then ponder why, during the Photoshopping process, it is a common practice to lighten the hue of the skin of a woman of color. (I'll give you a hint; racism is involved.)

This erroneous white standard of beauty creates additional hurdles for women of color to achieve body satisfaction.[i] If such a big part of achieving Effortless Perfection is looking a certain part, and subliminal messages are being sent that that part is white, we've got a mega problem. A racist agenda is being propagated here.

Jessie reflects, "My experiences in the beauty realm can be summed up in seven words: 'You are pretty for an Indian girl.'" This phrase, "pretty for a _____," is all too often used as a back-handed "compliment" for people of color and highlights the biases society holds about who "gets" to be beautiful, she explains. There's essentially an asterisk placed after the word "pretty" implying that, by default, women of color are not attractive. Commentary of this kind is disgusting and absurd, yet phrases such as these are used too often to be ignored.

Mia has similarly seen racial bias in regard to beauty impact both herself and her loved ones. She watched her older sister deal with body image issues in high school and college as a woman of color. Mia explains:

> *My sister did all her high school at a private school in Georgia, a state where, if I'm being honest, many private schools were created for the sole purpose of avoiding integration of Black and white students back in the day. So, they are still somewhat strongly segregated now and my sister struggled as one of the*

[i] I want to address the severity of these issues, but I also do not want to disrespectfully cross a line by speaking for a story that isn't fully mine to tell. To make up for any potential gaps in this chapter, I recommend reading Stephanie Covington Armstrong's *Not All Black Girls Know How to Eat: A Story of Bulimia* and Becky Thompson's *A Hunger So Wide and So Deep: A Multiracial View of Women's Eating Problems.*

only Black women at her school. Even though she was tall and thin, she still didn't feel like she fit the definition of femininity for that community.

It was not until her sister entered into college, where she became close friends with a large group of Black women, took classes on race and gender, and became strongly involved on campus, that she seemed to develop a stronger body confidence and feel more secure in her identity and her femininity.

For Mia, her insecurities center less on her body and more on her hair. She feels that "the whole natural hair movement has taken off and fought against the notion that Black hair in its natural state is 'unkempt.'" But she also notices that women in the Black community continue to face judgment when they don't take steps to chemically straighten their hair or otherwise change it from its natural state to fit into today's biased and prescribed standard of beauty.

Just look at the picture below showing what used to come up when Googling "unprofessional hairstyles for work" versus "professional hairstyles for work" before they addressed the algorithm issue.[4]

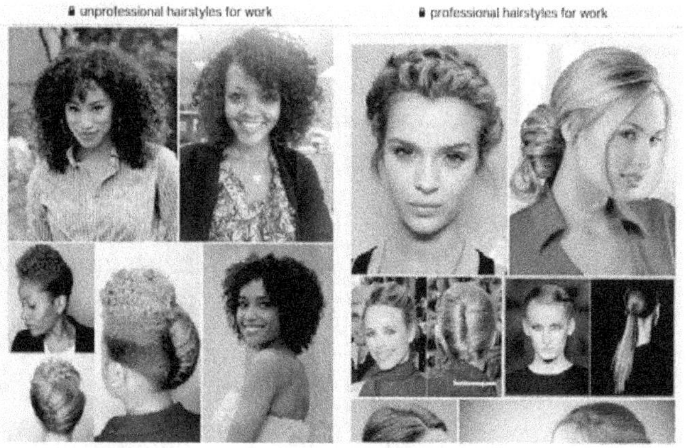

Though she embraces her hair now, when she was younger, the lack of understanding around "how Black hair works" and the way other students regarded her hair as "different" and "strange" made her feel alienated.

Representation matters because our self-concept is impacted by the images we see on a day-to-day basis. Katie affirms she "kind of didn't realize that [she] looked Hispanic or different than 'normal white people' when [she] was younger." She remembers always looking for a similar face in a TV show or magazine, but never really saw anyone with an "olive tone." Rarely, there would be an African American represented if the form of media was "trying to outwardly be diverse," but otherwise it was "always extremely blonde hair and blue eyes." She wondered where she fit in. Was she "in the middle" or was she "something entirely different?"

She adds that, now, she obviously knows that she is Latina, but her journey with making sense of her body has included some additional twists and turns: "I have curves, ya know? And it's interesting how, well, I guess a lot of people, guys especially, fetishize Hispanic and Latina women. There's this reinforcement of 'we want you to be this way, we don't like skinny girls, "ethnic" bodies are more beautiful,' but it's all sort of still about trying to fit me into a box and I'm not sure how I feel about it." Katie draws attention to the point that, while all women tend to be held to one overarching societal beauty standard depicted in dominant culture, they also feel pressure to simultaneously meet their community-specific beauty standards, which can sometimes even be contradictory.

Overall, the Effortless Perfection Myth often impacts individuals differently depending on their identity markers. Its stringent expectations are extremely difficult—sometimes even impossible—for all women to live up to, especially the projection of an "ideal" beauty that often discounts, or outright ignores, the countless manifestations of beauty that women of color represent. It is important to note the various different pressures women of all races and ethnicities face when attempting to live up to particular standards of beauty under the Effortless Perfection Myth because, while some of our struggles may differ, we are all fighting back against an issue that spouts from the same spring. To take down this issue, we must approach it from all angles and understand the different ways it impacts us all. We cannot afford to leave anyone behind.

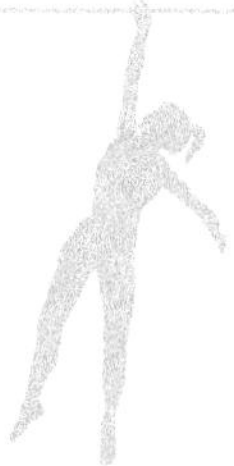

Chapter 25

More Than Just Looks

ONE OF THE MORE FRUSTRATING THINGS about struggling with disordered eating is how the disease is often written off as a superficial fixation all about looks. Disordered eating, as an issue, has been widely publicized. But the one-dimensional caricature that's been propagated along with that public service announcement has erroneously been that of a white upper-class sorority girl who was vain enough to get so caught up in her appearance that she just withered away. It's infuriating for those of us who know disordered eating does not discriminate—it impacts people of all races, socioeconomic statuses, social affiliations, and genders. And it's particularly infuriating for all those who have ever struggled with disordered eating to see our plight get written off as nothing more than a superficial desire to achieve the perfect "beach bod."

Disordered eating is a deeply emotional and symbolic behavior.

"I don't get it. *Why* am I doing this to myself?" I remember bawling to my psychologist in one of our first sessions. "I know it's hurting me. I've seen how it has the ability to take away my favorite parts of myself—my empathy, my ability to care about pretty much anything beyond this stupid fixation. It's like there's this bug in my brain controlling my thinking. Everyone keeps saying it's not about food, it's not how you look.... But I really wish it were those things. It would be so much easier that way to end this misery, to find a solution.... And if it's not those things, *what is my reason*? What could possibly be such a big deal that it would drive me to *this* extreme?"

When I first started therapy, I went in looking for a silver bullet. I was expecting a Freudian moment where my dark secret would be unveiled and I could be instantaneously cured. Instead, my psychologist patiently explained to me that there wasn't likely just one reason. Life comes with built-in pressures and stressors with which we all must deal and, in order to do so, we each develop our own personal coping strategies.

Some coping strategies are healthy (meditation, yoga, eating nutritiously). Some are not (drugs, alcohol, self-harm, excessive spending). Some start off healthy, but become unhealthy at their extremes (work, diet, exercise). I happened to fall into this last category.

"So, what you're saying," I processed out loud, "is that everything, all of it, *life,* is the reason I developed my eating disorder.... That it's all the complexities and uncertainties of my day-to-day, month-to-month life that have led me to engage in anorexia and overexercising because that's the system I've developed for coping with such things? But that by taking it to the extreme I have, it's now a negative instead of a positive. So, what was once a means of self-protection has gone awry, and transformed into a threat to my well-being...yes?"

"Bingo."

When I came forward for help with my eating disorder, I was given incredible support from concerned friends and family, as well as a dedicated team of professionals on my college campus ready to set me on a path toward recovery. It felt as though all these hands were being extended to hold me up and keep me steady as I wandered into what would no doubt prove to be difficult terrain.

That said, there were often times during the recovery process that I felt misunderstood—to the point it felt as though my struggles were being invalidated—because of the stereotypes surrounding the issue. Disordered eating often gets portrayed as a superficial, shallow habit having to do solely with looks when, in actuality, it's an addictive, all-consuming mental illness that develops from the desperate desire for a sense of safety and control in what can feel like an overwhelming world.

I had multiple epiphanies about the nature of my disorder in therapy. Some key ones I put together in a piece I wrote for the National Eating Disorders Association are:

- *Disordered eating is not so much a choice as a triggered response.* Those who are most impacted by the triggers don't tend to be the surface-level, image-obsessed people we get stereotyped as. Most often we are the ones I once heard an eating disorder specialist refer to as "porous," meaning we are sensitive to external vibes and the undertones of what hangs in the air. Porous individuals tend to internalize what everyone else is emitting—anxiety, social competition, anger, sadness, jealousy—into common spaces. We feel all these things and we feel them so intensely that we don't know what to do with it all. Overwhelmed, our brain kicks in with a coping mechanism (not unlike drugs, alcohol, or other addictive forms of release) as an escape.

- *Disordered eating is a distraction from the things that are actually scaring us.* We tell ourselves, "Once I lose these next five pounds, I will have what I need to be *happy*." Or "Only when the scale says this number will I know I'm truly *safe* from those trying to bully me and hurt me." Or "Only once I fit into that body-con dress will I feel like I *belong* in this campus culture." By taking our fears and—instead of allowing us to feel them—only focusing on losing weight as the *one* solution to *all* our problems, we are given a way to feel in control. Except that feeling of control doesn't come from actual control; it comes from being so distracted and detached that we become oblivious to reality. "The nature of obsession is that it protects you from the truth," writes self-help guru Geneen Roth.[1]

- *Our weight becomes symbolic and metaphoric.* "Thin" becomes synonymous in our minds with words and phrases like "protected," "strong," "admirable," "successful," and "in control." Meanwhile, "fat" becomes synonymous with words and phrases like "vulnerable," "weak," "failure," and "out of control." We have a hard time separating "thin" and "fat" from these words of greater consequence because they have been melded together out of fear—the kind of fear that reduces complexities of life into oversimplified concepts so they can feel manageable even when they aren't.

- *Weight is numerical and exact.* We know that if we eat X amount of food, and exercise Y amount, the scale should say roughly Z pounds. The definitive quality of that number, the sense of there being an equation behind it, and the belief that if I take one action then I can expect a certain result is addictive for those who feel too many aspects of their lives are unpredictable and unruly.

- *Disordered eating most often arises from emotional upheaval that has gone unexpressed or been invalidated.* (This links back to Chapter 15 on assertiveness and the importance of expressing things like pain and anger.) For example, there is disturbing incidence of sexual abuse in the backgrounds of women who exhibit the most extreme behaviors of disordered eating. Some may be trying to lose as much weight as possible to reject the feminine curves that would otherwise draw attention and make them potential objects of lust. Others may attempt to reject that kind of attention in the opposite way by gaining excessive amounts of weight. Manipulating their bodies in this way adds to their sense of security because it gives them a way to feel protected from being violated a second time. Their eating disorder may also be a form of protest against what happened to them.

Notice a trend with each of these key take-aways? Not a single one stops at just image or looks. Each one stretches into issues of control, fear, love, unmet need, and desire. There is immense complexity tied to disordered eating. Keep this in mind and be gentle with those struggling with this issue, whether that is someone you know or yourself.

The next logical progression after realizing that my eating disorder was a coping mechanism that had spiraled out of control was to figure out why I had been compelled to take my coping to such extremes. During therapy sessions, the culture of Effortless Perfection on campus came up time and time again as I discussed the increase in pressures and insecurities I experienced upon entering college. Sure, these things had been issues in high school, but definitely not to the same extreme. (Although disordered eating symptoms and attitudes may be established long before college, prevalence studies have revealed that disordered eating tends to peak in late adolescence and early adulthood—during the college years and slightly afterward.)[1]

In essence it was as though, as soon as I entered college, the accelerator got pressed down on everything. I had already been given reasons to question the mechanical soundness of my means of coping along the way. There were multiple warning signs I'd chosen to ignore in the heat of the college race: a noticeably wiggly axle, a signal blinking red on the dashboard for low tire pressure, an atypical breakdown over a statistics exam here, an overheated reaction from a misbegotten relationship there. We all experience different versions of these warning signs as women chasing Effortless Perfection in college.

So why do we keep going, engines revved, despite all the signs telling us there's a bigger issue at stake? What exactly is it about the Effortless Perfection Myth that is alluring enough to ensnare smart, capable, powerful young women and convince us to irrationally chase such painstaking extremes?

I think it's that, to a certain extent, we don't think we have a choice and our college environment often makes it hard to see any other possibilities. As time passes, we stop believing there's something wrong with the system for being so impossibly demanding and decide there must be something wrong with us for not being able to keep up.

Chapter 26

The Denial of Female Appetite

AS WE NOW KNOW, disordered eating is a symbolic behavior stemming from the desire to integrate the overwhelming complexities of life into a simplified system of concrete assumptions that feel more manageable. Unfortunately, the further this ill-fated coping mechanism spins out of control, the harder it becomes for us to differentiate our emotional needs from our physical needs.

For instance, a study of more than 900 girls in seventh to tenth grade found that "emotional deficits—particularly a failure to tell distressing feelings from one another and to control them—were found to be key among the factors leading to eating disorders." The researchers concluded that "these girls need to learn to identify their feelings and learn ways to soothe themselves or handle their relationships better, without turning to their maladaptive eating habits to do the job."[1]

Much like the girls in this study, many of today's collegiate women develop complicated relationships with food and body image because we feel the empty ache of the black hole that comes from chasing after Effortless Perfection and are confused as to what the source is. Consequently, we begin making misdirected attempts to soothe ourselves. We *physically* binge, stuffing food into our bodies, in an attempt to make ourselves feel more *emotionally* full. We *physically* purge, expelling food from our bodies, in an attempt to feel less *emotionally* weighed down.

With this in mind, let's pick apart the symbolism embedded within disordered eating from a different angle. First, we must recognize the way we, as a society, employ many of the same words to relate to our stomachs as we do to relate to our souls: "nourished," "famished," "fed," "full," "starved." This language overlap is no coincidence. There is a definite link between our physical and emotional selves.

Appetites exist in full circle. "Food is love...and love is sex, and sex is connection, and connection is food," author Caroline Knapp writes.[2] All these aspects of our multidimensional selves work in tandem, so it's difficult to suppress just one of them without suppressing all the others. It's best that each be given equal weight—celebrated in a way that is fair and undifferentiated—to keep the circle working. So what happens when young women are raised under an ideology that tells us to feed our souls, while starving our bodies?

A paralyzing negation takes place, that's what.

Society cannot teach women to physically shrink ourselves, and expect that this will not also be interpreted as an instruction to make ourselves smaller within all spaces we inhabit. By constantly sending messages to women about food—mainly diet, deprive, deny—society is subliminally messaging us to approach our entire lives according to this paradigm. And we are *listening*.

The runaway rate of disordered eating and its strong gender bias are proof of this. Nine out of ten individuals suffering from an eating disorder are females between the ages of twelve and twenty-five.[3] Furthermore, women in this age group are also three times more likely than men their age to engage in subthreshold levels of disordered eating (meaning that their behaviors fall on the disordered eating spectrum but are not so severe that they warrant a full-symptom diagnosis).[4] And why? *Because we are sent a different message from the one that is sent to young men about the overall acceptability of our appetites, both literally and metaphorically.* From physical hunger to sexual hunger to hunger for power and purpose, each of these receive drastically different reactions if expressed by a man versus by a woman (as already laid out in the chapters focused on confidence and assertiveness).

While "the hunger of boys [is] so vivid and clear, expected, accepted as fact," the hunger of girls is regarded as "dangerous and secretive and fraught with consequence," Knapp argues.[5] For instance, a guy can pile food on his lunch tray and scarf it down without commentary, while a girl can't do the same without hearing a line like "You're eating *all* that?" Studies show that parents urge their sons to eat regardless of weight while only urging daughters to eat if exceptionally skinny.[6] And in 2014, parents asked Google, "Is my daughter overweight?" roughly 70 percent more than "Is my son overweight?"[7]

As a result of the mixed messages we receive about the acceptability of our bodily hungers, young women don't always feel we have permission to act upon the wider range of emotional hungers we naturally experience. Only a select few are okay, and even then they must be carefully managed. Thus, in today's age, we may feel more comfortable using our voices to say, "I'm going to go after this" or "I want to accomplish that," but we still don't know how to use those same voices to say, "I'm starving. Society is placing expectations on me that are really hurting me, and I don't know how to tell you because I don't want to let you down."

Instead, many of us find ourselves using our bodies to express that discontent and need indirectly. We've noticed how much attention our bodies receive, so we try to harness that and make some use of it. Our bodies become our mouthpiece, the vehicle for a whole range of expression we don't feel we have the medium to express in any other way. For instance, I used my eating disorder as a way of communicating to all the pressures and expectations coming at me from all angles: *I don't know what you want from me, so I'm just going to make myself as small as possible until there's nothing left for you to pick apart.* It took me far too long to recognize that, with this approach, I was only hurting myself.

My relationship with disordered eating and Effortless Perfection was not unlike being with an abusive partner. It was familiar, comforting, and reassuring, always there and always willing to pull me back into its tight grip. But in order to receive its "love," I also had to put up with its bullying. I had to endure constantly being told I was fat and ugly. I obeyed the demands imposed upon me for the promise that, eventually—once I'd made myself perfect enough, once my body no longer showed any signs of excess—the voices telling me I wasn't enough would shut up.

The reality is that the voices never shut up so long as you feed into them. They will take every inch they are given, and the more you give, the louder they become.

In her book *Perfect Girls, Starving Daughters*, Courtney Martin illustrates how perfectionism leads women to despise the parts of ourselves with needs, mainly our hungers and discomforts. She asserts that, under the pressure to perform and perform perfectly, our basic needs come to seem like burdens holding us back rather than normal healthy functions. Because we find it so hard to control and deny ourselves of those needs, we begin to resent much of what makes us human.

Martin fleshes out this theory by outlining two dichotomous identities women create for themselves in their attempts to live up to the standard of perfection. First, there is the "perfect girl"; she is what the outside world sees and she embodies all that we want to be known as. She has no needs. She just perfectly performs and effortlessly delivers. Then, there is the "starving daughter"; she is made up of the leftovers. She embodies the individual's guilt, shame, jealousy, anxiety, and insecurity—all the needs the "perfect girl" has but is not allowed to show.

Martin explains, "Beneath the façade [of the perfect girl] is the daughter—starving for attention and recognition, starving to justify her own existence."[8] But this part of us annoys us as it "slows us down" and "embarrasses us." This second half is the half that doubts our ability to handle things, who feels emotions like fear and loneliness. It's this second half, we tell ourselves, that's to blame every time we "drink too much" or "cry too loud" or "seek comfort in cookies, coffee ice cream and warm bread—transgressions that make [our perfect self] angry."[9]

We think that by giving a second persona the parts of us that feel feelings we don't like and struggle with struggles we don't want to be real, and then excommunicating that second persona, we can live the Effortlessly Perfect lives we've always dreamed could be ours. But this schizophrenic split only turns us into our own worst enemies.

We cannot dissect ourselves into good and bad parts, strengths and weaknesses. Often these pieces of ourselves are so intertwined that they are one and the same. We are made up of singular traits with positive and negative outcomes depending on the context. For instance, in one context, my ADHD is a central part of my creativity and my goofy persona—two of my favorite things about myself. In another context, my ADHD is also the source of great frustration because the excitement I feel inside in social contexts often causes me to unintentionally interrupt others (a lot). The energy that builds, the drive within me to put my thoughts and feelings out into the world in expressive ways, is a source of both pride and shame in my life. While I can try my best to elevate the positives and soften the negatives, I cannot cut them apart and keep one while discarding the other.

The same is true of empathy. Your empathy might be central to the strength of your relationships with others—a main source of joy in your life. But, in another context, your empathy might also be the source of a great deal of pain and anxiety when the people or things you care for are threatened or put in harm's way. Your empathy in this second scenario might push you to make rash decisions, to be overprotective and obsessive. But you cannot cut these outcomes apart so as to feel only half of what your empathy brings you.

One cannot be without the other. We are both. To reject the Effortless Perfection Myth, we must invite our "starving daughter" to become one with our "perfect girl" again. We must thread ourselves back together.

Chapter 27

Recovery and Embodiment

RECOVERY FROM AN EATING DISORDER can be incredibly difficult because, without our disorder, we often don't fully know who we are. Particularly for those struggling with anorexia, being skinny often comes to feel like our defining feature, if not our full identity. That potential loss of identity (even if only temporary until life becomes refocused as we get better) is not to be underestimated or disregarded, because the disruption of that sense of self can make those of us actively trying to get better feel incredibly anxious, fearful, and vulnerable.

To make matters worse, for many of us this disorder is the only coping mechanism we ever developed. Without other coping skills at our disposal, recovery can mean a terrifying transition full of loss and agitation, while also having no means of managing our emotions. We feel exposed and achingly raw.

Recovering from an eating disorder is "an inherently murky and nonlinear process" wherein consistent motivation is difficult to sustain, progress is hard to quantify, and relapse can come in all sorts of deceptive, alternative forms.[1] Those with eating disorders can't just give up food the way a recovering alcoholic or drug addict might give up the source of their addiction. We can't simply refrain from situations putting us in the way of temptation—that's what our addiction was all about to begin with. Now we must learn to be okay with the opposite, to place the thing that has come to symbolize our fears and strike at our anxieties right under our very noses.

Such a challenge often requires help from a therapist and a nutritionist, someone to hold us accountable. Until we are willing to commit to such things, it's difficult to truly get better.

When I first recognized that I had a problem, like many others before me I chose to do nothing about it because, deep down, I wasn't ready to get better. I still depended on my disorder too much—it was my strongest source of reassurance in the face of the Effortless Perfection Myth and there wasn't much that was going to change my mind or behavior. Not the programs hosted every now and then by my school, not the voiced concern of friends and family members,[i] not even the threatening health statistics listing the potential hazards of self-starvation and overexercise:

- Increased risk of heart failure due to the eating away of muscle tissue necessary to maintain heart rate and blood pressure
- Reduction of bone density and increased risk of osteoporosis, resulting in dry and brittle bones that break more easily
- Severe dehydration leading to potential kidney failure
- Extreme fatigue, fainting, and overall weakness
- Hair loss and dry skin
- Intolerance to cold
- Loss of sex drive
- Loss of period and, if prolonged, loss of fertility
- Heightened risk of depression

I knew I was at risk. I was even experiencing some of the less extreme symptoms already, but I still didn't care because, at the end of the

[i] Nevertheless, these efforts were all still very helpful in that they planted the seeds that brought me to ask for help sooner rather than later when I finally came to terms with the full extent of my problem.

day, *I was skinny*. The chaos and pain I had falsely come to believe were waiting for me on the other side of "skinny" were far more concerning to me than the physical consequences about which I'd read.

So, regardless of the shocking headlines and terrifying statistics—like "a review of nearly fifty years of research confirms that anorexia nervosa has the highest mortality rate of any psychiatric disorder"[ii2] or "for females between fifteen to twenty-four years old who suffer from anorexia nervosa, the mortality rate associated with the illness is twelve times higher than the death rate of all other causes of death"[3]—I was going to keep doing what I was doing. As far as I was concerned, the National Eating Disorders Association could report whatever it wanted. I was good. I was fine. My fixation wasn't an issue; it was propelling me closer and closer to Effortless Perfection, closer and closer to the life I'd been chasing.

Too many people spend too much of their lives thinking that their issues with food and body image are "not bad enough" to invest in changing. They wait until hitting rock bottom. I can identify. I did exactly that. But what everyone needs to understand is that "not bad enough" is still far from "good," and it usually only gets worse.

When I took my first steps onto campus, I already had some of the habits and coping mechanisms of disordered eating ingrained in me. I reached for them consciously and unconsciously and, though the unhealthy thinking was a part of my daily thoughts, I still had somewhat of a separateness from it.

[ii] Official death rates are hard to ascertain because anorexia victims often die through proximate causes like heart attacks and suicide (disordered eating and depression often occur in tandem). Five to 10 percent of those who suffer from anorexia will die within ten years of developing the disease.

I wish I hadn't pushed off confronting my problem, waiting instead for the terrifying moment down the road when I realized that nothing seemed to matter to me as much as the treadmill and my running shoes, the only routine that still ensured a sense of security within me. I'd clung to this shred of security as my body dysmorphia convinced me the scale was wrong and the mirror couldn't be trusted. Regardless of what everyone said, I was certain I was getting bigger and bigger—expanding, overflowing every day.

I had yet to understand that this wasn't just some battle I was fighting inside my head; it was seeping into every aspect of my life, pushing me into physical and mental isolation.

The physical isolation was the result of my fear of social situations involving food, which made me tempted to avoid them all together. I didn't realize this also often meant memories lost. Going to grab frozen yogurt with a friend, indulging in drinks at a sorority mixer—these are the little moments that make up one's college memories. I was en route to missing too many of them on purpose, all in a panicked effort to avoid calories.

The mental isolation was even worse, especially when it reached its extreme. Even when surrounded by friends and family, I wasn't actually there. I was stuck in my head because it's impossible to be fully present in a moment when all you can think about is the fact that you are hungry, when the only thing your focus is going toward is not eating a second slice of pizza.

People would tell stories, recall memories that I was physically but not mentally present for, pushing me to realize how absent I had been. I was forced to understand how my obsessive thoughts had placed me in a different world from the one in which these memories had taken place, the world in which I would have been able to share in these stories, to laugh and cry and be a part of something. My inability to feel, to connect, hit me in a way that was unbearably dehumanizing. Only then did I realize all that I had traded for the chance to be the kind of skinny I thought Effortless Perfection required.

One of the most difficult parts of recovery is mourning all that has been lost in the years battling the disease. I'd let my pursuit of "skinny" sink deeply into my heart instead of reserving my heart for more important things. This was devastating. In my grief, I realized I wanted nothing more than to love this whole life harder, to connect again with all the people in it and love them to the absolute best of my ability. Simultaneously, I recognized just how far away I was from being able to truly do so, due to my disorder, and it ripped me to pieces.

How did I get here? I questioned myself again and again. *How did I allow myself to become so broken?*

I imagine my feelings at this point were somewhat similar to those of a person realizing they've spent the last five years in a cult. I'd picked up on some questionable things here and there, until I finally pieced together that I was stuck inside a lie. In order to make it out, I had to break down that lie to reveal each of its inaccuracies and then I had to let that lie go.

This necessity became most clear to me when attending a group therapy session in which we all went around the circle and answered a question: What does your eating disorder promise you? The answers ranged from "It promises me my family won't have to worry about me," to "It promises me safety from being sexually assaulted again." I listened to the others in the room respond and I listened to my own response, which came from some deep-down place inside I did not often let myself visit, and realized that the reasons we were doing what we were doing had absolutely nothing to do with being thin!

Once that much was clear, I delved deeper and deeper into what the incredibly loaded word "thin" actually meant to me. I asked myself: Is the behavior I'm engaging in actually going to get me what I want, or do I have some wires crossed here? The obvious truth forced me to confront that my brain had been hijacked by a lie that had spurred a delusional obsession. I needed to take back the reins.

At its core, recovering from an eating disorder—and Effortless Perfection for that matter—is about stripping away all the inaccuracies, misunderstandings, and untruths involved in your belief of who you are and why you do the things you do. You must look closely at each of the things you consider to be the facts of your life with fresh eyes and determine which ones are wolves in sheep's clothing. Then you must untangle those falsehoods from your obsessive behaviors until they are no longer obsessive because they have been sucked dry of the false promises that made them so addictive in the first place.

Once you've banished your eating disorder's lies from your brain, the final step to recovery is embodiment. In short, you must convince your mind that your body is now a safe place to live and invite it back inside.

Your mind will be timid at first, suspicious. It will remember the bashing and regulating and manipulating that used to define its relationship with this body. But your mind will also remember the value of having a true home in which to reside. The hope it has long held onto that this might once again be possible will allow the two to rebuild that home in a healthier way.

Rebuilding this relationship absolutely must be a core tenet of modern-day feminism. As author Rachel Simmons asserts, "The work of empowering girls cannot live above the neck." We can toil away helping young women with their self-esteem, confidence, and assertiveness on an intellectual level, but until they feel those things down into their fingertips and toes, we've failed them.

We need women's growing sense of power and agency to include our corporeal beings. In her book *On Female Body Experience,* Iris Marion Young writes:

> *[Women] often experience our bodies as a fragile encumbrance, rather than the medium for the enactment of our aims. We feel as though we must have our attention directed upon our bodies to make sure they are doing what we wish them to do, rather than paying attention to what we want to do through our bodies.*[4]

Socialization has caused us to see our bodies as passive sites that are acted *upon* instead of active sites that we can utilize to further our personal and political interests.

To fully embrace embodiment, we must stop thinking of our bodies as encumbrances. For the longest time, I tried to convince myself, "I am not my body, I am not my body," as a way of overcoming my body image issues. I blamed my own flesh as the source of my sorrows, rather than all the messages intent on convincing me my body was something of which to be ashamed.

Until one day I realized what was going on. I realized that by repeating that phrase—"I am not my body"—over and over as a way of distancing myself from the flesh I'd come to see as a major source of shame, I was surrendering even further to the socialization and ideology that had caused my body dysmorphia and eating disorder in the first place.

I finally understood why I'd never been able to fully accept that mantra. I needed to recognize the power this corporeal vessel held and take it back for myself. Enough was enough. It was time to stand up to the media, advertising, and other sexist institutions trying to take ownership of my body. And so my mantra flipped and became: *I AM my body. I am not THEIR body.*

This distinction is important to understand because it is only through our bodies that we get to experience life. You are the only person on the planet who will ever experience first-hand pleasure from your own eye slits and through the touch receptors on your fingertips. Your body is for you. Think of what it does for you.

It's time to stop rejecting our bodies and start recognizing them as worthy places to live. It's time to start treating our bodies like they belong to someone we love, to claim them back for ourselves. As actress Salma Hayek once said, "People often say that beauty is in the eye of the beholder, and I say the most liberating thing about beauty is realizing you are the beholder."

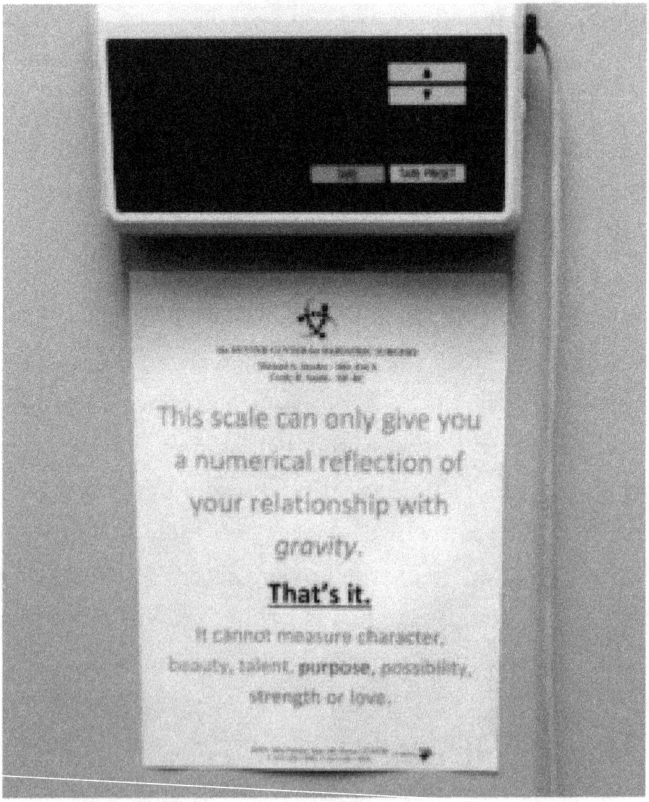

Something to remember the next time you choose to step on a scale.[5]
If you are concerned that you may be struggling with disordered eating, I encourage you to take this online screening: www.nationaleatingdisorders.org/online-eating-disorder-screening.

Section V

Putting Ourselves Out There

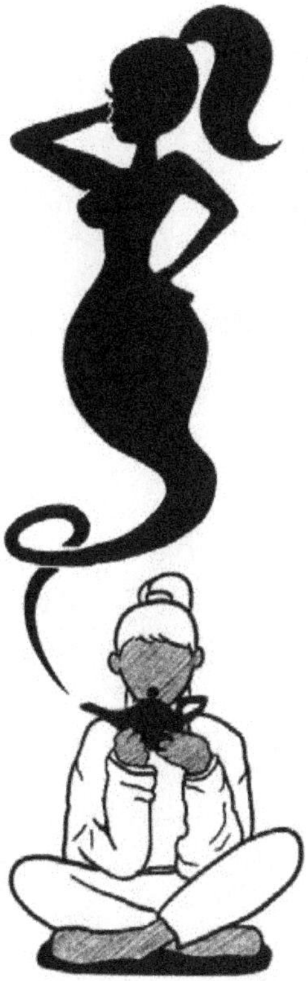

Chapter 28
The Ambiguous Hookup

OF ALL THE CONTRADICTORY EXPECTATIONS placed on young women today, the sexual ones are by far the most confusing, especially upon entering college. Effortless Perfection in high school is, for the most part, about playing the part of the "good girl," as discussed in Chapter 6. Thus, the so-called "proper" way to be sexual as a young woman from the ages of fifteen to eighteen is pretty much not to be sexual at all unless one is in a long-standing relationship, and even then it's meant to be kept as private and on the down-low as possible. This setup does not exactly give us much wiggle room to explore in ways that we may find empowering, but at the *very* least it is straightforward.

Then college comes along and the game completely changes. Effortless Perfection is no longer just about being the "good girl" when it comes to the sexual realm—a realm that is suddenly receiving greater emphasis in our lives than ever before. Effortless Perfection is now also simultaneously about embodying an image of sexual prowess and empowerment inside and outside of a relationship.

Obviously, there is an inherent contradiction in this situation. Such empowerment logically includes the power to decide whether, when, and how often to be sexual. But how are collegiate women supposed to figure out what we really want when we are busy fending off all the strong opinions everyone else is hurling at us? How are we supposed to manage the expectation of sexual prowess, while also managing the expectation of continued "innocence"?

Even if we were to decide we wanted to be in a relationship before engaging in sexual activity, the college-dating scene isn't exactly a wonderland when it comes to looking for a committed romantic partner. With the advent of hookup culture, the spaces in which female undergrads form relationships have become increasingly difficult to navigate. The new pressures existing today—such as the pressure on guys to meet hookup quotas, and the pressure on girls to ramp up our sex appeal and lower our inhibitions—make relationship choices more difficult. What are we to do?

The general consensus is that hooking up is designed to avoid the emotional "entanglement" of a relationship. The term "hookup" is kept intentionally ambiguous so as to imply that anything from a make-out session to full-on intercourse may have taken place. In *The End of Sex*, Donna Freitas writes, "What define[s] a hookup more than the sex itself [is] the perception of its meaning (or lack thereof) by both participating parties."[1] She believes it is less about a physical exchange or even about sexual gratification, especially for women, and more about fulfilling a social expectation.

The social contract one mutely agrees to before a hookup commences is that both parties should be able to walk away from the experience as if it never occurred. Any disappointment caused if the engagement proves to be a one-time thing is the fault of the person who was hoping or expecting more, because grounds for that kind of attachment are nowhere in the hookup contract. Such attitudes and behaviors have brought much disdain and even alarm from previous generations, as has been showcased by numerous publications labeling it a sort of moral panic. In the opinion of Boston College professor Kerry Cronin, "Hookup culture is about the commodification of myself; buying and selling myself to make myself less lonely, while at the same time making myself lonelier in the process."[2] (She is definitely not a fan of this phenomenon!)

I think the conversation needs to be switched from whether hookup culture is a good thing or a bad thing to a discussion of how to navigate it. Because, at the end of the day, it's less something college students have chosen for themselves and more something inherited from their slightly elder peers, who, in turn, inherited it from their own slightly elder peers. Opting out is complicated, and straight-out rejecting hookup culture can feel like a decision to miss out on a major part of what's "supposed" to make college fun.

Collegiate women should have the freedom to choose how we engage within the hookup culture, as long as we remain honest with ourselves about what it is we are looking to get out of it. Which is precisely where I think the trouble starts. As female undergrads, we aren't being all that honest with ourselves a good deal of the time because we are allowing the groupthink mentality surrounding hookup culture—the same groupthink mentality surrounding Effortless Perfection—to have too great an impact on our choices.

In the pursuit of greater honesty, we need to be checking in with ourselves more often and asking questions that challenge the dominant narrative, like: Is this truly fulfilling? For all or for some? In what contexts and under what conditions? What are the driving forces behind it all? What apparent norms am I willing to accept, and which am I not?

Chapter 29

All in the Subtext

IN HIS *NEW YORK TIMES* ARTICLE "The End of Courtship," Alex Williams tries to peg the origin of hookup culture. He theorizes that it is the result of old-fashioned dating being "subverted" by new forms of connecting and communicating:

> *Traditional courtship—picking up the telephone and asking someone on a date—required courage, strategic planning and a considerable investment of ego (by telephone, rejection stings). Not so with texting, e-mail, Twitter or other forms of "asynchronous communication," as techies call it. In the context of dating, it removes much of the need for charm; it's more like dropping a line in the water and hoping for a nibble.*[1]

Fair enough. Considering how the majority of my relationships began in college, there was definitely a lot of "Hey, I'm going to be at ____ place tonight. Feel free to come." A guy texts a girl to stop by a party his fraternity is hosting; if she doesn't come, he doesn't have to feel rejected because he never fully put himself out there. A girl messages a guy she likes asking what he's up to that night; if he invites her over to hang with his friends, it may be code that he is also interested…or it could mean nothing. It is all one big play on potential: Where could this lead? Is this actually something?

Hookup culture makes it harder to admit one's feelings up front without coming off as trying too hard. It's yet another place to showcase Effortless Perfection by acting nonchalant about romantic prospects, like you can't be bothered to care too much or actively pursue somebody because you have so many theoretical options available in hookup land that you don't have time to catch feelings.

As a result, more happens in the subtext. Nobody is forthright. Nobody shows the cards they are holding. A kiss doesn't have to mean anything, so what used to be a way of communicating "I like you" can now be reframed as a drunken blip. The same thing goes for sex; it could mean something, or then again, nothing at all. So we now see more of these loose "relationships" that fade in and fade out without a definitive beginning or end.

Jordana Narin, a student at Columbia University and 2015 winner of the *New York Times'* Modern Love College Essay Contest, captures this disconnect in her piece "No Labels, No Drama, Right?" She describes how she has had feelings for a guy since their first kiss four years ago, but still hasn't actually told him about those feelings. She can't get over the possibility of being with him, but she also senses it's too late to say anything:

> *I'm told my generation will be remembered for our callous commitments and rudimentary romances. We hook up. We sext. We swipe right. All the while, we avoid labels and try to bury our emotions. We aren't supposed to want anything serious; not now, anyway. But a void is created when we refrain from telling it like it is, from allowing ourselves to feel how we feel. And in that unoccupied space, we're dangerously free to create our own realities.*
>
> *. . . Women today have more power. We don't crave attachment to just one man. We keep our options open. We're in control.*
>
> *. . . But are we?*[22]

She laments that, while she and this guy have been involved with each other for multiple years, the two of them are "technically nothing" since they never put a label on their relationship. Is she truly "empowered" if she remains stuck in a pattern of "brood[ing]," unable to share her feelings? Could her options "possibly be any more closed"? Without that label to connect them, she has no way to justify her ongoing feelings and he has no obligation to acknowledge those ongoing feelings either.

Narin wonders how accurate it is no claim "no labels means no drama." Her piece demonstrates that, in being so hesitant to define or at least acknowledge outright our relationships in the context of hookup culture, we are participating in a type of deviation from them. Too often it is the unlabeled person, the one we never really had in the first place, whom we still secretly hope, against all odds, might be "The One."

There's no closure, and no definitive way of asking for any, especially because the culture of Effortless Perfection assumes that the relationship/hookup world should be navigated with ease or, more accurately, with a blasé attitude that suggests the only way to triumph is to be the one in the pairing who cares the least. Showing one's cards would mean taking off one's mask and allowing oneself to be vulnerable, which is the number one thing Effortless Perfection forbids.

Unfortunately, this dynamic often leads to subpar results, particularly since those looking for intimacy have been known to engage in hookup culture as an ill-fated shortcut to the closeness they crave. For example, in a 2018 Me Too Monologue[i], an anonymous female student paints the scene of her typical hookup experience. A guy approaches

[i] See Chapter 43 for more information on this student-led theatre production focused on issues of race, gender, and sexuality at Duke.

her at a bar. She initially feels good about herself and excited about the interaction taking place. She agrees to go home with him after an hour or so of flirting and dancing. Once back at his room, the interaction is still very much consensual—he asks if she wants to keep going and she candidly says yes.

Hooking up feels good for a bit until she finds herself unable to think about anything other than whether or not she is living up to his expectations. He seems "infinitely more comfortable in [this] state" because, while "he doesn't give a fuck how he looks," she finds herself worrying about whether she remembered to shave, appears bloated, or "look[s] half as good as his favorite porn star or his ex-girlfriend." She has to remind herself that she "wanted this, too."[3] Then, at last, the moment arrives that she has really been waiting for all along:

> *It's finally over and you just lay there with your head on his chest. I guess it was actually okay. Maybe it was worth it.*
>
> *But no less than five minutes later, he gets up.... He says he's "not really into girls sleeping over." You look at him with slightly wounded eyes, but say nothing. "It's just a personal thing," he says. "It's not you."*
>
> *And [suddenly] you're* that *girl. That girl who thinks she can hang and is chill but... he doesn't really want you there. He's talking to you because he has to and you want to leave, but god dammit the only reason you are there is for the intimacy, for the conversation, for the feeling of being close to someone who for a second is validating every part of you.*
>
> *And somehow, you've deluded yourself into thinking it's that guy before you. Scrolling through his Instagram feed instead of looking at you adoringly, admiring your beauty, and talking about your guys' lives. So what can you do?*[4]

Our protagonist is overcome with a sense of rejection at the very moment she was expecting to receive the intimacy she so craved. She must quickly "feign a detachment that no part of [her] feels" and gather up her pride along with her clothes before making a quick exit.[5]

Deep down, she had hoped that agreeing to get to know each other better physically would also mean an opportunity to get to know each other better emotionally. Like 43 percent of women who engage in hookups, her ideal outcome for this encounter would have been that it eventually led to a traditionally romantic relationship.[6] Her hopeful expectations for and the actual endpoint of this interaction are sorrowfully misaligned, and she feels stupid for believing this could have led her anywhere else but out the door of this guy's dorm room, alone, at two in the morning.

However, she's not alone in these feelings of shame and embarrassment. According to a study in the *Journal of Sex Research* authored by five Loyola Marymount psychologists, female undergrads are twice as likely as their male counterparts to experience distress after hookups. When asked, "Have you ever hooked up with someone and afterward had the feeling that the person respected you less because you hooked up with him/her," 54 percent of women said yes, while only 22 percent of men said yes.[7]

College psychologist Dr. Gary Glass hypothesizes that this kind of confused and disenchanted feeling is experienced at much higher frequency than it once was. He explains that, previously, "conventional wisdom" for a man who wanted to get a woman to sleep with him was to "just tell her 'I love you.'" In such a scenario, if she did end up sleeping with him and was then ignored or mistreated, she had every reason to feel slighted. She could call out the guy for behaving with "conscious and intentional dishonesty."[8]

However, Dr. Glass has noticed that the typical narrative he hears from disheartened female undergrads during counseling sessions has changed. With the advent of hookup culture, he explains, "Using somebody for sex no longer relies on the lie of 'I love you' because it became more efficient to deliver the lie, 'It doesn't matter to you whether I have genuine feelings for you.'" Furthermore, this "lie" is now delivered, not from one individual to another, but to and by the collective long before an actual encounter even takes place.[9]

Dr. Glass believes this setup is actually more toxic than the original because those who feel cheated can't call foul or hold the other person accountable. It is no longer "clear and socially acknowledged" that a person who has sex with you and then doesn't call back or acknowledge you afterward lacks integrity. The prevailing thought is: *So what if they used you for sex? In hookup culture you are both supposed to be using each other for sex—that's the point.*

An even worse outcome occurs when the assertion "It doesn't matter whether I have feelings for you" is extended further into "It does not matter that I disrespect you."[10] Charlotte reflects that this kind of mindset led her into some tenuous and twisted "relationships" in college:

> *As a freshman and sophomore, I just wanted that love from another person so badly that I misplaced, or misinterpreted, what it really means to be loved. I accepted some very false versions of love. I would get treated like shit all the time and think, well at least he calls me once a week, at least he finds me attractive...and all the other bad things that came along with those positives were just, you know, part of what it was to receive love in my mind.*

She continued to give a great deal of herself for very little in return until her junior year when she "completely flip-flopped." Suddenly, she found herself rejecting the idea of love entirely because the version of it she had been accepting for the last two years had been incredibly painful.

Admittedly, Charlotte is on one end of the spectrum. At the other end, Jordan admits to playing along with the norms implemented by hookup culture without feeling jaded or thinking twice. She says that even if a guy did express genuine interest in her from the start—opting to soberly ask her out on a date instead of drunkenly inviting her back to his room—she would likely be "weirded out," not because that isn't what she wants, but because hookup culture reinforces the notion that we should not be forthright with our emotions.

The relationship timeline that Jordan is used to begins with a drunken hookup, potentially followed by more drunken hookups, followed by sober interactions, followed by deeper conversation and personal connection, followed by revealing interest in and feelings for one another. To her, and to many of her peers, this is the natural progression of intimacy. Thus, her initial reaction at the start of any potential relationship with a guy is to always think "this is just physical," until given a concrete reason to think otherwise. That way, if things don't lead to a legitimate relationship, she can at least relish the social capital gained through hooking up, bringing her one step closer to achieving Effortless Perfection.

Chapter 30

Uneven Power Dynamics

THE YEAR BEFORE I ARRIVED at my university, a twenty-year-long tradition of "progressives" had just come to an end. Progressives were parties wherein select sorority girls were chosen to serve as "hosts" for potential pledges that fraternities were hoping to draw.[i] The night of the event, there would be a series of rooms with different themes in which the girls would wait for freshmen boys. The boys, blindfolded and often in little more than their boxers, would be led through this maze of dark rooms where the girls, who were almost always quite drunk themselves, would "haze" them—allegedly performing acts such as straddling them dominatrix-like, calling them babies and forcing them to suck on bottles full of alcohol, and pouring chocolate syrup and whipped cream on one another and having the guys lick it off.[1]

While some may argue that this could be a powerful experience for these women being given a somewhat dominant role over the guys entering the room, the party was still designed by and for

[i] The tradition ended after a student-group put together a panel of Greek leaders and Women's Center administrators to speak at an open forum entitled "Perspectives on Progressives." Though there were panelists arguing both for and against these parties, the conversation circled around issues of "sexual assault, female empowerment, and social hierarchy." A petition to end the "particularly coercive, negative type of progressive" was circulated, with criticism and backlash continuing until these kinds of parties were banned entirely.

men. Women could only participate if they were willing to act out one very exhibitionist form of sexuality. Their sex appeal was their most valuable asset and they wouldn't be invited if they weren't willing to put it to use.

While progressives are a more extreme example than the typical college party, similar dynamics are constantly at work to a certain extent. Many parties are designed to endorse sexual promiscuity on behalf of women. Typical themes involve the same kinds of role-play pairings one might find in porn: Execs and Secs, Superheroes and Supersluts, CEOs and Office Hos, GI Joes and Army Hos, Workout Bros and Yoga Hos, Santa and His Reindeer Ho Ho Hos. Note that the guy is always in a position of power and authority, while the girl plays a more submissive, dependent role. Oh and, also, we get called hos a lot. (Shout-out to the one fraternity that humorously challenged the norm with the theme "CEOs and Women We Respect a Lot.")

On the next page are two examples from my freshman year of the kind of listserv emails that fraternities sent out to selections of the female population to promote their parties. Though most of these emails didn't tend to be nearly this overtly sexist (or racist or homophobic), it wasn't not outside the norm for those elements to be included.

A *Chronicle* article on the topic notes that the emails are "products of an arms race among fraternities who use crude humor to catch the attention of their social circles" and "that competitiveness drives people to push the limits."[2] Regardless of the excuses, at their core these emails send out the message: *This is what we think of our female peers. This is how we feel comfortable addressing you.* And that dynamic is more than a little disheartening.

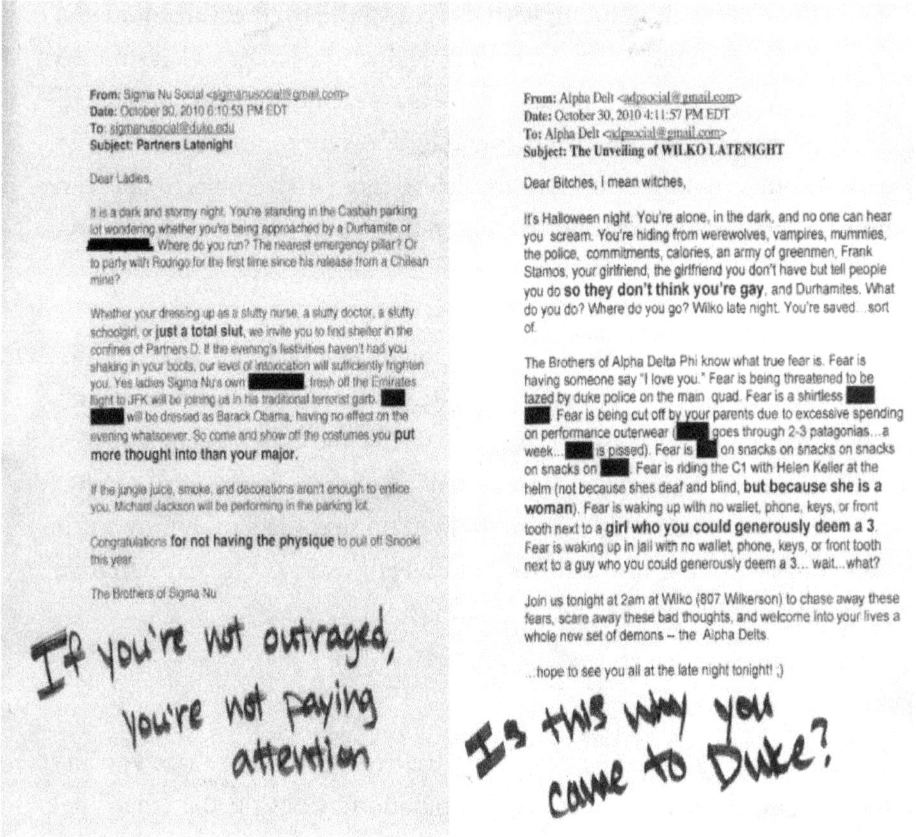

From: Sigma Nu Social <sigmanusocial@gmail.com>
Date: October 30, 2010 6:10:53 PM EDT
To: sigmanusocial@duke.edu
Subject: Partners Latenight

Dear Ladies,

It is a dark and stormy night. You're standing in the Casbah parking lot wondering whether you're being approached by a Durhamite or [redacted]. Where do you run? The nearest emergency pillar? Or to party with Rodrigo for the first time since his release from a Chilean mine?

Whether your dressing up as a slutty nurse, a slutty doctor, a slutty schoolgirl, or **just a total slut**, we invite you to find shelter in the confines of Partners D. If the evening's festivities haven't had you shaking in your boots, our level of intoxication will sufficiently frighten you. Yes ladies Sigma Nu's own [redacted], fresh off the Emirates flight to JFK will be joining us in his traditional terrorist garb. [redacted] will be dressed as Barack Obama, having no effect on the evening whatsoever. So come and show off the costumes you **put more thought into than your major.**

If the jungle juice, smoke, and decorations aren't enough to entice you, Michael Jackson will be performing in the parking lot.

Congratulations **for not having the physique** to pull off Snooki this year.

The Brothers of Sigma Nu

From: Alpha Delt <adpsocial@gmail.com>
Date: October 30, 2010 4:11:57 PM EDT
To: Alpha Delt <adpsocial@gmail.com>
Subject: The Unveiling of WILKO LATENIGHT

Dear Bitches, I mean witches,

It's Halloween night. You're alone, in the dark, and no one can hear you scream. You're hiding from werewolves, vampires, mummies, the police, commitments, calories, an army of greenmen, Frank Stamos, your girlfriend, the girlfriend you don't have but tell people you do **so they don't think you're gay**, and Durhamites. What do you do? Where do you go? Wilko late night. You're saved... sort of.

The Brothers of Alpha Delta Phi know what true fear is. Fear is having someone say "I love you." Fear is being threatened to be tazed by duke police on the main quad. Fear is a shirtless [redacted]. Fear is being cut off by your parents due to excessive spending on performance outerwear ([redacted] goes through 2-3 patagonias...a week... [redacted] is pissed). Fear is [redacted] on snacks on snacks on snacks on snacks on [redacted]. Fear is riding the C1 with Helen Keller at the helm (not because shes deaf and blind, **but because she is a woman**). Fear is waking up with no wallet, phone, keys, or front tooth next to a **girl who you could generously deem a 3**. Fear is waking up in jail with no wallet, phone, keys, or front tooth next to a guy who you could generously deem a 3... wait...what?

Join us tonight at 2am at Wilko (807 Wilkerson) to chase away these fears, scare away these bad thoughts, and welcome into your lives a whole new set of demons – the Alpha Delts.

...hope to see you all at the late night tonight! ;)

[3]

These two emails, in particular, created a backlash on campus from undergrad women who printed them out and posted them across campus with commentary like "If you're not outraged, you're not paying attention."

Customary themes at frat parties like Catholic Schoolgirls and Playboys often call for us to dress provocatively, and many of us do so willingly—excited to have an excuse to show off some skin and feel sexy, relishing the attention we can draw. The Effortlessly Perfect girl is expected to so in the name of empowerment, as if to say, *I'm taking control of how I look and the statement I'm making.*[4]

It's a way of responding with dissent to the overbearing, outdated virginity movement, a way of rebelling against the unfair, old-fashioned dichotomy that frames men and women as "conqueror and conquered" or "free agent and desperate girlfriend."[5] We want to assert our right to express our agency, as opposed to feeling like passive objects that can only be acted upon. We want to reclaim the spaces for sexual expression that have long been denied to us, and this seems like the best way to do that.

Still, there are plenty who aren't convinced. Donna Lisker, former associate vice provost for undergraduate education at Duke, maintains, "They've gotten this message from the media and other places that part of being a modern woman is sort of playing with your sexuality.... What they don't necessarily get...is that you put on that Playboy-bunny outfit and you're stepping into a history of objectification."[6] Is that narrative really the one we want to be reinforcing?

In 2006, *Rolling Stone* reporter Janet Reitman came to Duke with intentions of capturing the student population's vibes on the (then) recent lacrosse scandal.[ii] What she came away with was an overall report on the university's hookup culture, mostly from the female perspective. Her lengthy exposé—which could honestly describe any number of schools minus the specifics—initially makes it appear as though women are the ones fueling the hookup culture. A male student is quoted saying that guys do not have to go "all out" to get girls to go home with them the way they would if they were out at, say, a club in New York City. "There's a kind of a mutual acceptance that stuff can happen in one night, on your way back from [the bar]," he explains.[7]

[ii] Three members of the Duke lacrosse team were falsely accused of rape by Crystal Magnum, a Black student at North Carolina Central University who worked as a dancer and stripper.

However, as the article progresses and more of the situational complexities are revealed, it becomes clearer that this role in the hook-up culture is one that most undergrad women feel pushed to play rather than one they gallantly chose for themselves. As the female interviewees let down their guard, contradictions and conflictions in their feelings are exposed. "Girls reduce themselves a lot here in order to be able to have the sexual freedom that I think they *don't* have by doing that," one wearily confesses.[8]

It's hard not to cringe at the rather unflattering image Reitman's article relays of the lives of many college women. Lisker is quoted saying, "Our undergraduate women…are the best of the best. They're so smart, so driven, top of their class, student-government presidents, lettered in every sport,"[9] yet, when it comes to their personal lives, she feels they seem to forget all that in their efforts to meet the social rules set by male peers. She laments, "[Men] throw the parties, they create the expectations, they create the standards, and these women—these incredibly smart women—on some level, being accepted by their peers is so important that they put aside their own values and standards. They dumb it down."[10] What's worse, the female undergrads often don't even realize they are doing it.

Early on in Reitman's article, sophomore Naomi reports feeling certain that there's more "sexual equality" now than ever before and that the issue should no longer really be up for debate since "an even sexual playing field is a given…or at least should be."[11] Later in the article, though, Naomi makes a completely antithetical comment: "It's our decision if we're going to allow ourselves to be subjected to negative treatment. It's all framed by the way girls behave."[12] The juxtaposition of these sentiments reveals that Naomi is holding two contradictory beliefs in her head. She is claiming complete sexual equality, while also giving women the lower hand by implying that if we receive negative judgment for our sexual choices (the kind men almost never have to deal with, mind you) then *we* are the ones to blame.

This impossible situation ties back to the Effortless Perfection Myth because, just as it's impossible to approximate perfection without effort, it's impossible to feel empowered while accepting this double standard. Female undergrads bend over backward to make this impossible hookup culture logic seem natural and easy-breezy, but I don't know if we are really fooling anybody.

Chapter 31

The "Lucky-to-Be-with-Him" Mentality

IN MY EYES, the most eye-opening part of Janet Reitman's previously mentioned *Rolling Stone* article is the dialogue captured between two fourth-year women, Allison and Kasey. Allison begins by confessing that she has done things completely against her values in order to make a relationship work with a guy in a "high-profile" fraternity, all out of "a constant fear of losing." Kasey concurs, "When you're in a relationship with somebody, especially with somebody in the frat scene, you're *lucky to be with him*" [emphasis mine]. No matter how beautiful or smart the girl, she contends it is "never the other way around."[1]

Allison then lets herself get emotional: "I found myself falling into this thing.... It made me very uncomfortable and unhappy, because it's not a way to live. But if I didn't do these things and he broke up with me for some reason, two days from now he'd have somebody else. That's just how it works."[2]

What's devastating about this exchange, from a cultural standpoint, is the way in which these women so clearly feel shortchanged, while passively accepting their lot as just the way things are. The passage is drenched with a tone of dissatisfaction. In college, I wanted to believe just as much as Reitman's interviewees that women could feel as empowered as men in today's current hookup culture. I was just as reluctant as they were to admit this is usually not the truth, especially on a campus where the Effortless Perfection Myth—along with its dependence on hooking up as a form of social capital—runs so rampant.

The things Allison confesses about her controlling, double-standard-riddled relationship are hard to hear. Harder yet is being able to personally relate to her and the *lucky-to-be-with-him* mentality. To a certain extent, I have known the feeling, too.

The first guy I was really into in college wrote me a long, hand-written letter on Valentine's Day, a very sweet gesture, after about a month and a half of getting to know each other. The letter ended with him saying he could see us becoming exclusive. The next day, when I showed excitement over this, he countered by saying something along the lines of "Don't get your hopes up too much; I'm not making any promises." I tried to shake off the comment and pretend not to feel offended, but there was an uncomfortable undertone suggesting that I had to be something really incredible to draw him away from all these theoretical options awaiting him in hookup land. He made me feel as if I was the only one between us who had to prove themselves.

This was the first of many times I would encounter the lucky-to-be-with-him mentality. A discussion with a close friend revealed a more extreme example. She had been in a budding relationship with a guy and was so used to the whole "lucky" mentality that, when he first told her he loved her, she found herself just staring back at him, flab-bergasted. She was so taken off-guard that she had to fumble for words when he went on to ask if she felt the same way. She explained to me, "I had been so set on just trying to 'land' him and keep him, I hadn't even begun to consider whether or not I *loved* him." We both agreed (with no shortage of embarrassment) that in the context of the campus hookup culture, we had come to operate in a way where we didn't give complete thought to whether or not a guy was truly the right fit for us until we were sure he was going to stay! Only once that pressure was off could we honestly evaluate.

Call us crazy, but our reasons for operating this way were somewhat justified. Jon Birger explains in his book *Date-Onomics* that, when it comes to collegiate dating, the numbers are lopsided in favor of men. As a financial and tech journalist, Birger has concluded after "a combination of demographics, game theory, and number crunching" that single, college-educated, heterosexual women really do have it harder in this realm.[3] We are now enrolling in college at higher rates; for every four female college grads there are three male college grads nationwide. This skewing is only projected to increase; the U.S. Department of Education expects the ratio to reach three women for every two men by 2023. This gender imbalance has been linked to decreased traditional dating and promotion of casual sex because men feel comfortable being more selective with whom they choose to become exclusive. Thus, they tend to spend more time "shopping around" and delaying relationships because, in crude market terms, the supply is higher than the demand.[4]

A study by Dr. Jeremy Eucker of University of North Carolina at Chapel Hill and Dr. Mark Regnerus of the University of Texas at Austin called "BARE MARKET: Campus Sex Ratios, Romantic Relationships, and Sexual Behavior" found that "a more sexually permissive climate" (i.e. one where hookup culture is prevalent) is correlated with "less favorable treatment of women on the part of men," who are more likely to regard them as "sex objects."[5]

Jane has definitely noticed this issue on Virginia Tech's campus. She notes, "In the college frat and sorority scene," the lucky-to-be-with-him mentality "is *definitely* a thing. Sororities are so big, it's like there's a revolving door of girls for the guys." She recalls multiple situations where friends who had "had a thing" with a fraternity guy learned "sometimes even just a day or two after it ended" that he was already with someone new. As a result, many felt discarded and as though they "totally lacked control" in determining the outcome of their love lives in an environment where it's typically up to the guy to "decide what you are" or "DTR" (define the relationship).

This is particularly rough when considering how the culture of Effortless Perfection is in many ways about maintaining control—control over your academic success and future career prospects, control over your body image, and control over your desirability. The truly Effortlessly Perfect girl should be able to get whoever she wants whenever she wants. She has, in theory, "earned" that desire and romantic interest by molding herself into the perfect catch, so the way hookup culture so clearly robs her of that control she's jumping through all these hoops for can be jarring and demoralizing.

Melissa believes this lack of control leads to scenarios where, because the girl feels more replaceable, she is often the one who has to concede more to make the relationship work. In fact, numerous interviewees thought that, as a result of the imbalance caused by this setup, they were often made to feel like a nag when asking for common courtesy from their partners. More than a handful of my interviewees reflected with regret on the ways they had allowed themselves to be treated in past college relationships. Michelle at Duke notes, "When I first met the guy I'm with now, I would often thank him for doing basic things that should really be expected in a relationship and he'd be so confused, like, 'Why are you thanking me for following a baseline of respect?'"

While Michelle personally feels she has come a long way in pushing back against the mentality that Effortless Perfection and hookup culture primed her to accept, it doesn't take much for old anxieties to resurface in her current relationship. She admits, "I still find myself getting nervous he's just going to call it off suddenly. If I don't hear from him for a couple days, I panic that something has changed because those were the only signs I was given before." She knows that these fears are somewhat irrational, but, at the same time, these fears have been reinforced multiple times by those she has dated in the past. A great deal of her current behavior is still motivated by not wanting to "scare off" the person she is dating by asking for "too much." The lucky-to-be-with-him mentality has made it hard for her to feel secure in her relationships and she doubts that feeling will ever fully fade.

Personally, my biggest strategy for pushing back against the lucky-to-be-with-him mentality is to remind myself of a line from my favorite book (and movie) *The Perks of Being a Wallflower:* "We accept the love we think we deserve." One of my hardest, proudest college moments was telling a guy with whom I was involved that I had worked far too hard on my personal sense of self-love to let him continue to treat me the way he was treating me. I gave him an ultimatum that I knew would most likely lead to a breakup, asking him to step up or step out. He stepped out. As badly as I wanted the relationship to work and as lucky as I felt to be with him, I moved through my conflicted feelings by reminding myself that not standing up and saying I needed more than what he was giving me would mean that, somewhere in my gut, I felt this subpar "affection" was the kind of love I deserved. And I knew better.

Chapter 32
Sexual Entitlement

THERE IS A FCKH8 CAMPAIGN Instagram post that reads, "'Slut' is attacking women for their right to say yes. 'Friend zone' is attacking women for their right to say no. And 'bitch' is attacking women for their right to call you on it." I appreciate the post because it validates the anger I feel about the kinds of negative experiences women often face when choosing to engage in collegiate hookup culture. Just thinking about them makes my blood boil, especially when it comes to issues of intimate justice and sexual entitlement.

"Intimate justice" is a term coined by Sara McClelland of the University of Michigan to address the ways in which sex has personal and political implications that are connected to issues like inequality, power, violence, and mental and physical health.[1] Intimate justice asks questions like: Are both partners entitled to enjoy this experience? Is there a primary beneficiary? Are levels of expected satisfaction similar?[2]

The unofficial answers to these questions on so many American college campuses are a shot to the heart. McClelland's extensive studies show that when women engage in sexual activity they tend to "use the other person's pleasure as the yardstick for their satisfaction, whereas guys use their own pleasure as that yardstick."[3] Women tend to put their partners' desires before their own, thinking, "If they are pleased, then I'm pleased."[4] As an unfortunate extension of this, women are four times more willing than men to engage in sexual activity they don't like or want, such as oral and anal sex, to please or appease partners.[5] And that's where our people-pleasing tendencies can lead us into particularly dicey waters.

"This was absolutely the case for my first college relationship," reflects a Northwestern student who has asked not to be named—even with a pseudonym—due to the private nature of her account. She describes a dynamic wherein her boyfriend at the time pretty much demanded certain things from her sexually and she felt immense pressure to oblige. He'd also do things like ask to "just cuddle" and then inevitably start touching her in ways that "we both knew was more than a cuddle" to try to get her to cave. She can see now that his unrelenting behavior was inappropriate, but in the moment, she wasn't able to recognize this because it "didn't feel like he was being outwardly vindictive."

Lorelei Simpson Rowe, a clinical psychologist at Southern Methodist University who trains women on refusal skills, notes that scenarios leading to sexual violation and assault tend to involve plenty of "guilt-inducing tactics" like persuading and pleading, often combined with complimenting and flattering. Such actions can make a partner feel like the one in control of what's happening, when they are actually having power exerted over them by being made to feel uncomfortable and as though they are causing the other person distress.

Because of the subtlety of these tactics, "You see a lot of self-questioning among girls, 'Am I reading this right?' 'Did he actually say that?' 'Did he actually mean that?' Dr. Simpson Rowe explains. This is why such scenarios can feel so "gray," despite the fact that the language and behavior used to work out a "yes" is typically intentionally manipulative.[6]

The Northwestern student previously discussed really struggled with the "gray-ness" of her situation with her then-boyfriend. Her mindset became "I'm physically capable of doing this for you, not that

I want to do it, but apparently these are your needs." Meanwhile, her desires were treated as an afterthought at best. She reflects:

> *I know I should feel more comfortable advocating for myself and feel more entitled to physical relationships wherein the guy feels a responsibility to make sure I am comfortable and at ease while, you know, I'm making my body totally vulnerable in front of him, and where communication should feel natural, but right now that feels like a tall order. Like I know those guys are out there…but, at the same time, where the hell are they?!*

On one hand, she knows that a truly healthy relationship requires both partners to pay close attention to each other's boundaries and genuinely care about not crossing them. On the other hand, she feels hookup culture reinforces the notion that getting physical is now expected to be the first step of entering into a relationship, which fetters her propensity to set clear boundaries for herself.

At first, she justified the situation with her ex by rationalizing that all relationships require a bit of compromise. But she now knows in her heart that no relationship should require the kind of compromise in which one partner must disassociate from their own body in order to be able to please the other partner.

In her book *Dilemmas of Desire,* developmental psychologist Deborah Tolman explains the disconcerting aspects created by such a dynamic, since entering into the sexual world without being led by one's own sexual feelings puts girls "at risk."[7] The resulting disconnect with our bodies makes us especially vulnerable to traumatic sexual interactions because "when a girl does not know what her own feelings are, when she disconnects [or disassociates] from what is happening in her own body, she then becomes especially vulnerable to the power of others' feelings as well as to what others say she does and does not want to feel."[8] Such a dynamic begs the question: if you don't know what you *do* want, how are you supposed to know what you *don't* want?

Agency relies on being in touch with one's own desires. But multiple aspects of our collegiate hookup culture make it difficult for women to expect and experience embodied desire and feel comfortable determining the course their sexual interactions take. For instance, many girls' first sexual encounters are with older guys who already have experience, leading them to look to these older guys to show them how sex works and what to expect. (Even if it's not with an older guy, the expectation is typically that he has more of an idea about what he's doing.) What many young women learn under this power dynamic is notably from a male-centric viewpoint that is less inclined to take their female needs and desires into account.

Furthermore, many feel afraid to express their desires outright because, as author Chimamanda Ngozi Adichie explains in her TED Talk "We Should All Be Feminists": "We teach girls shame. Close your legs, cover yourself—we make them feel as though being born female they're already guilty of something. And so, girls grow up to be women who cannot say they have desire. They grow up to be women who silence themselves. They grow up to be women who cannot say what they truly think."[9]

Is it any wonder young men define bad sex as failing to meet orgasm, while young women define bad sex with words like "depressing," "humiliating," and "degrading"? Is it any wonder the largest survey on American sexual behavior ever conducted found young women reporting pain in their sexual encounters 30 percent of the time?[10] Certainly this cannot be what intimate justice looks like.

Not even close. Intimate justice demands that young women experience their sexuality as a form of physical pleasure or self-expression rather than a performance or an award to be won. It recognizes, in the words of Caroline Knapp, that "the ability to say yes is not the same as the ability to say *yes, with him but not with him*, or *yes, like this but not like that.*"[11]

We are far from reaching these requirements on today's college campuses.

These kinds of uneven power dynamics reinforced by hookup culture are only exacerbated by the way guys are often given greater control in the Greek collegiate social scene. Due to a stipulation where sororities are not allowed to provide alcohol at any social events unless hosted at a physical bar with licensed bartenders, fraternities essentially become the sole "suppliers" of alcohol since they are not barred by any such rule.[12] Thus, they play a greater role in deciding what the social world will look like because most events occur on their turf, since they are the only ones with permission to provide a key ingredient.

"Guys create the social spaces for the most part and girls just have to hope they will be invited," notes Michelle. The need to bid for an invite can affect the way women dress and carry themselves because there is a sense that, if they want to get invited back, they need to make themselves as appealing to their hosts as possible.

While the Effortlessly Perfect woman is expected not only to accept this dynamic, but also work it to her advantage with ease, reality reveals the opposite outcome is more likely. Michelle notices that college girls sometimes experience a kind of "quiet desperation" to find a guy to hook up with, or possibly date if it's in the cards (there's that lucky-to-be-with-him mentality again), because it ensures a more stable social life. By way of example, Michelle recalls multiple girl friends who were hooking up with or dating men all in the same fraternity and how, if she didn't "have a guy" in that fraternity or didn't know how to "act like 'one of the guys' to get invited," being part of that scene was simply not an option. Thus, not having some sort of a loose relationship with a guy in that fraternity meant she would not able to hang out with her own friends in their most common social space.

This kind of environment only serves to further reinforce a culture of sexual entitlement. A 2014 *Chronicle* article called "Entitled Men and Guilty Women" powerfully highlights this issue. Author Nicholas Russell Pollack begins, "Let me ask female students an absurd question: Do you feel that men have a right to your body?"[13] After supposing most would find such a question offensive, and rightly so, he asks the reader to consider a comment a female friend of his recently made to him: "Well whatever, it's just oral anyway. We weren't that drunk, and it's not like we were going to have sex, and I wanted to call it a night."

Upon hearing his friend make this statement, Pollack pushed back. Was she suggesting that leaving the guy sexually wanting would have been "improper" or "misleading"? Had the guy somehow intimidated her?

"Oh no," she replied, "I just...I would have felt guilty I guess."[14]

Guilty. Reluctant to disappoint or offend. Pollack wondered where this deep-seated feeling of "obligation" to please the guy who had been "courting" her came from. As he did, it dawned on him that she was not his first female friend to have made this kind of remark; in fact, if he thought about it, the collegiate women he knew were making these kinds of comments "with horrifying frequency."

Horrifying indeed when one considers the underlying assumption in such a statement that, if a girl does not want to have sex or linger, the reasonable course of action is to "blow the guy in relatively short order" and leave. Such a logic implies one critical assumption, Pollack notes—namely that "the guy must be satisfied before the girl may leave."

Pollack remains puzzled until imagining himself as the female in the situation. He invites the reader to do the same, to plop themselves into the shoes of a first-year girl who gets noticed by a fraternity brother and invited to a social event as a date. In the scenario, "sparks don't fly" but the guy is "nice enough" and the evening is enjoyable. Perhaps dinner and drinks were paid for ahead of time and, as a freshman new to college, you are grateful to have had the opportunity to mix with a new potential social circle. As the evening winds down:

> *[Y]ou find yourself alone with your host. The drink has worn off. You are lucid, not aroused by any means, but the guy feels differently. Desire clouds his eyes, plain to see. And you begin to feel a dilemma: If you should thank him for the evening, excuse yourself and leave without further ado—will he take offense? Will he feel slighted, cheated somehow? Will he give his group a bad account of the night, shattering your hopes of [hanging out with his social circle again]? Will you garner a reputation for being cold and distant so soon in your [college] career? These questions run through your mind, provoking other questions. What is a kiss, really? What is a couple of minutes of canoodling in the scheme of things? Will you even recall these minutes, come next week? A kiss and a feel, and everyone wins!*[15]

Such questions feel natural in a way, but what we are also seeing here is the perpetuation of a sexual entitlement that is profoundly dangerous.

A recent United Nations report studying gender-based violence found that rape is "most commonly motivated by a sense of sexual entitlement."[16] If female undergrads themselves are unconsciously validating such attitudes, then who is to say sexual predators will not continue to intentionally abuse their male privilege to pressure those vulnerable to this frame of thought?

Dr. Gary Glass notes that between his confidential one-on-one counseling sessions and the various collective student retreats and forums he moderates, "there are repetitive themes of entitlement in the stories that are told."[17] These stories typically suggest that "sex is 'a given' [and] that sexual access is a default reality, in spite of many efforts on campus to combat sexual objectification, harassment, and rape."[18]

The most common manifestations of sexual entitlement that Dr. Glass tends to hear about include these presumptions:

- When a girl refuses intercourse, she should "at least" provide oral sex as a consolation.
- When a girl accepts an invitation to a date function or other exclusive event, she is also nonverbally agreeing to the socially enforced expectation that she will get physically intimate with the guy extending the invite.
- When a girl dances in a risqué or flirtatious manner with a guy for an extended portion of the night, her body language is consenting to sexual activity that may occur later that night.[19]

Such requests and assumptions are uncomfortable for women to navigate, particularly for first- and second-year women, who have less footing in the existing social system. For instance, Katie admits, "In a way, when you are at a party and a guy tries to hook up with you, you may not be totally into it, but you kinda feel like 'Well, maybe I should' because the attitude at a frat party is like, if you aren't here to do that than what are you here for?" She acknowledges that this dynamic is "troubling and kind of hard to deal with," but she can't help but "just feel this way all the time."

Brooke at Georgetown reports that, for her personally, there have "absolutely been certain cases" when she's run into these kinds of uneven power dynamics, but that it was "highly dependent upon who the guy was." Thankfully, she has had way more positive experiences where her male partner was "very conscious about making sure I was comfortable, checking in with me, really invested in me enjoying myself."

However, she also reflects that she is pretty avid about cutting things off with guys who are likely to be too sexually aggressive before things progress.

That said, she concedes it is "not always so easy to tell" and pretty much every girl she knows, including herself, has experienced some form of sexually aggressive or manipulative behavior. She feels somewhat lucky that her worst experience was going back with a guy who proceeded to forcefully push her head down to his crotch while they were making out in bed.

She reflects: "The expectation was just so clearly that because I had gone back with him that I was going to do this and he didn't need to do anything for me first or even ask me if I was okay with doing this for him. His action of pushing my head was like a way of saying 'This is what's expected of you and I don't know why you aren't doing this on your own.'" Luckily, she had enough experience to know that this was not acceptable behavior and was "able to get herself out of there," but recognizes that not all women always feel comfortable asserting themselves in the same way due to the uneven power dynamics at play.

The topic of Effortless Perfection may seem somewhat disconnected from this issue, but it is indeed embedded in how college women deal with the tricky matter of rape culture and the threat of sexual assault.

A major element of maintaining a front of Effortless Perfection is projecting that everything is always under control. Whether dealing with the workload from our classes or the expectations placed upon us by hookup culture, we expect ourselves to know what to do. Admitting that there was a moment we weren't in control, admitting someone else got the better of us, admitting we have experienced a trauma that took away our sense of agency and our right to choose—those things don't fit the image we are trying to project.

We want to be strong. We want the world to think of us as superwomen. So we hide our wounds from view and we try to stitch ourselves back together with unsteady hands. But the truth is that we never do as good a job as could be done if we sought help from others, whether from friends, family, or professionals. For many, remaining in denial feels easier. Keeping that burden a secret feels like a good way of protecting our loved ones from the truth, and maybe also ourselves to an extent.

Yet it is in this way we end up isolating ourselves from one another, when we could be comforting, supporting, and banding together with those who have struggled and are struggling with the same experiences. Instead, we could be sharing enough of our own vulnerabilities that others don't feel the need to hide their own. And what kind of a world could we make if we didn't feel the need to hide anymore?

Chapter 33
Nice Girl Syndrome

REMEMBER BACK IN CHAPTER 15 when we discussed how girls are commonly socialized to put likeability before all else? Not only are gender roles and restrictions disadvantageous in this way, but they can be downright dangerous.

Psychologist Beverly Engel warns in her book *The Nice Girl Syndrome* that it is possible for women to be "too nice for their own good," especially when it gets in the way of upholding their own values and setting personal boundaries.[1] She explains, "[B]ecause nice girls tend to be focused outside of themselves—helping others, worrying about not hurting others' feelings—they don't focus enough attention on protecting themselves, their feelings, and their very safety."[2] There is a downside to the selflessness so venerated in females.

Melissa confirms that when she was younger she felt obligated to do favors for others, even if she knew they would never return those favors. In retrospect, she reflects there were certain situations where she was "not even being 'nice' anymore," she was "just being pushed around."

Katie also noticed herself falling into a somewhat similar trap in high school. "I tried so hard to be a 'nice girl,' but it got me in bad situations because I would sacrifice myself to help others with situations that were so much bigger than the two of us," she notes. "I've heard it said you shouldn't 'burn yourself to keep others warm' and totally agree and am happy I dropped the act when I did." She recognizes how unhealthy that behavior was and has worked hard to get to a place where she's less afraid to say "no" or "I can't."

Being compliant and doing as told without question, passively letting things happen rather than risking argument, letting others get their way instead of vocalizing resentment—these often feel like the "proper" ways to act as women because we are often seen as peacekeepers in our families and communities. We are often the ones expected to neutralize conflict, to back down to keep our relationships even-keeled. "I'm usually the first to apologize or take ownership of things," notes Cole, an undergrad at New York University.

We don't often consider how being "too nice" and overly invested in the good of the whole is something that can make us more open to manipulation. By being too eager to please, too willing to bend over backward to avoid conflict, women send a strong message to those who may wish to take advantage of our willingness to compromise and accommodate and forgive. That unfortunate message is: "My need to be seen as nice (or sweet or innocent) is more powerful than my instinct to protect myself."[3]

Engel warns that these are the same habits and behaviors that make women prone to things like abusive relationships, sexual assault, harassment, and other serious consequences if left unchecked. And yet, these are exactly the behaviors that studies show women are expected to perform, and receive criticism for not fulfilling. We are in a serious bind.

One of the most important lessons I learned as an undergrad was this: *It's not rude to stand up to someone who is making you uncomfortable. You do not have to cater to them.* This may seem obvious when put in such terms, but my overwhelming desire to placate and keep everyone happy made it hard for me to fully internalize this concept right away. It took me a good number of bad situations to fully realize what was meant by it and how to act on it, particularly within the hookup culture I was thrown into in college—a culture I was both somewhat excited for, but also terrified of and extremely ill-prepared to handle.

When speaking with various upper-level women in college, a strong message rings clear. Many of us are not proud of the things we've had to experience in the process of getting to where we are now in our willingness to be assertive in unpleasant and demeaning situations. Because of this, many agree that these experiences are just as important to share with our peers as the academic- and career-oriented stories of disadvantage discussed earlier. For only in sharing our stories can we open ourselves to each other's support and become part of a larger, more powerful narrative. We have the ability to use our stories to spark the outrage needed to make things different, instead of sweeping them under the rug and into the dark—leaving our sisters and ourselves to experience them, and the pain that accompanies them, in isolation.

The Effortless Perfection Myth and the "good girl" persona it pushes us to adopt will want to make excuses like *he was drunk* or *I was being too passive because I didn't want to cause conflict; it's really my fault.* (Note: neither of these justifications is valid.) But when we swallow the blame and remain silent, we surrender our power to do or change anything. Silence does not have the power to erase.

Tina at Duke knows all too well that silence cannot erase the memory of being groped, hands literally in her bra, off the side of the dance floor of a venue because she didn't know how to tell the guy to stop. She didn't think she was allowed to tell him no, or know how to assert herself within the power dynamic created by their age difference (he was two years older). She thought she liked him and didn't yet know if this was just "normal college behavior" she was supposed to let happen, regardless of how she felt about it.

Silence also cannot erase her memory of the frat bro who decided five minutes into meeting her at a party that it would be appropriate to take her to the dance floor and attempt to finger her up her skirt even though they had never said more than three words to each other. Or the guy she said no to multiple times before being made to feel so uncomfortable, so ashamed that she was not meeting his sexual expectations, that she ended up going further than she wanted.[i]

These experiences all had an impact at one point or another on how Tina saw herself and her place in the college world. "All those times I was in those coercive situations—the reason I didn't just leave, didn't just walk away and get out of there—was because *I honestly didn't feel like that was something I was allowed to do*," Tina says. She sees now she had been conditioned to feel like something was owed on her part, like she was required to still act courteously, to people-please, and to avoid making any trouble.

She had believed she was doing what anyone else in her shoes would have done. She hadn't yet started talking to other girls about these kinds of situations, so she didn't know what she was and was not allowed to be outraged by. She didn't have the shared space to put her own experiences into the context of everyone else's.

Like many of my interviewees, Tina now mourns for her younger, more naive self who had to go through such things and for the many young women like her harboring these and even deeper wounds. Even

[i] It goes without saying that the large majority of my interviewees shared similar experiences, but I have chosen to discuss only Tina's for several reasons. 1) Sexual harassment and assault are issues that require full books to adequately address. While these issues fall under the wide purview of problems associated with the Effortless Perfection Myth, there are other resources already on the market that do this topic the full justice it deserves. I recommend *The Hunting Ground* documentary and the book *We Believe You: Survivors of Campus Sexual Assault Speak Out* as places to start. 2) I want to demonstrate the impact of these issues through the eyes of a singular female student. These are all the experiences of just *one* undergrad—an undergrad who did not drink until her senior year or have a single one-night stand while in college. If this is what just one of my interviewees discussed experiencing, imagine the multitude of painful stories I received from all my interviewees collectively.

more painful, she claims, is considering that she feels extremely *lucky* that these are the worst experiences she's had.

She is one of many collegiate women who has had to learn the hard way that mastering Effortless Perfection and gaining love and approval by playing the "good girl" will not protect us from harm. If anything, it may make us more prone to harm.

We must internalize: *It is not rude to stand up to someone who is making you feel uncomfortable.* We must tell those who haven't had to be jaded in these kinds of ways yet: *You are allowed to just get up and leave. You are allowed to tell someone to fuck off if they are blatantly disrespecting you. You are allowed. It is your right to assert your own willpower, to protect yourself by putting yourself first.*

Furthermore, we must recognize that this is not just a personal issue, it is a political one. Instead of maintaining this silence about our negative sexual experiences, we should be sharing our stories of struggle with each other. Jordan asserts that this kind of collective action supports one of the initial tenets of feminism:

> *[M]ost times girls reflect on a personal experience like that and think, "Oh, that's private," or "It was just this one specific circumstance with all these irregular factors involved," or "I don't want to talk about it because it's uncomfortable. . . ." But then you hear others tell similar stories and you realize that your experience isn't the only one and there are actually many. It's not just some personal thing that happened to you, it's something that happened to all these people and is something that needs to be fixed on a nationwide, even worldwide scale. It's like, holy shit,* this matters. *This thing that I thought was just me is everyone, and all women, and the only way we can change it is if we realize how far it spans.*

Jordan also notes that this perspective helps individuals to rid themselves of self-blame for the negative experiences that have left them feeling hurt or victimized. They better understand that what they are going through is bigger than just them, because there is actually a structural issue at hand.

The issues we face as collegiate women struggling against the Effortless Perfection Myth and its sexist expectations desperately need to be inserted into the public sphere, for it is only there that they can be discussed, examined, and solved. Our personal problems are valid, and they are often manifestations of bigger political injustices. Thus, to confront our own personal problems is a tremendously political act and also, ultimately, a collective act.

Chapter 34

The Norms of Hookup Culture

AS FAR AS I CAN TELL, college campuses are full of first-year women with bright eyes and eager smiles, ready to see for themselves what the hookup hype is all about. They've been sold the idea that "empowered women" should be able to "manage their romantic lives like savvy headhunters" by utilizing the "temporary intimacy" of a hookup while not taking any focus away from studies and job searches.[1]

Some even argue that hooking up has become the convenient replacement for dating, particularly on high-achieving campuses (the kind where Effortless Perfection especially flourishes), because students don't have the time or energy to invest in full-fledged relationships. The pressure to achieve, to maintain a perfect GPA and land the perfect internship, all while keeping up with numerous extracurriculars and *still* finding time to go to the gym to work out and bars to be social—when that pressure gets too strong, it's overwhelming.

With a limited number of hours in each day to fulfill these demands on our time, having a significant other we know also deserves adequate attention can leave one feeling even more stressed about not being able to do it all. With such little room for error, distractions become increasingly frustrating. Some women don't want to deal with the emotional investment or time commitment of anything more than the occasional hookup, and that's more than okay.

Still, from what I've personally experienced and heard most of my peers express, most female undergrads do not harbor positive feelings toward the hookup situation on their campuses. For every eager freshman, there seems to be an equal number of jaded upperclassmen, hurt by the hookup culture without fully understanding why or feeling they have anyone to blame but themselves.

Hookup culture, when combined with the dynamics of Effortless Perfection urging undergrads to hide their true feelings and compete against one another for academic and social capital, imposes some very harmful norms. Surprise, surprise.

The dominant narrative on college campuses leads many to believe that everyone engages in hookup culture and something is wrong with us if we personally don't also enjoy it. While this prevailing belief is not actually true on several accounts (more on this in Chapter 36), it does lead many of us to accept the following:

- *Norm 1:* We are acculturated to regard sex as a casual, no-big-deal experience and to think of those who want things like love and commitment to happen first as naive and setting themselves up for disappointment. Hooking up is supposed to be about maximum gratification with minimum risk. Since emotional attachment is risky, we are meant to numb our feelings in order to participate without getting hurt.[2]
- *Norm 2:* We learn to put out signals that portray us as wanting something that's often different from what we actually desire (i.e. we act like we are cool with just a hookup when many of us want connection beyond that). This is an ill-fated habit because once an interaction is grounded in a particular expectation, it's much harder to change the direction of where things are going.
- *Norm 3:* Since the name of the game is quantity over quality,

the emphasis is on pursuing more of what is new rather than maintaining what is worth still having or even growing. We are pushed to seek pleasure (immediate and fleeting) rather than contentedness (requiring patience, but longer-lasting).

- *Norm 4:* We treat hooking up as a means of gaining proof of social status. This is done in a way that frames what is otherwise an intimate interaction as a triumph rather than a connection. Thus, fellow participants are often regarded as conquests rather than partners.
- *Norm 5:* The system tends to exploit younger female students by emphasizing higher status for older male peers, while discarding older female students as less desirable.[3] This also tends to make it so that older men who have more sexual experience and feel more in control within the hookup culture are paired with younger women who have less sexual experience and feel less confident making their own rules and guiding the interaction down the path with which they are most comfortable. It's usually left to the guy to determine what a hookup looks like.

Obviously, all of these norms can have negative effects on women. Some may feel fine accepting them, but many don't.

Anne from Wake Forest summarizes, "I think that for those who are skilled at compartmentalizing their feelings, who don't want progression, they just want that release or quick burst of feeling, then hookup culture has pros for them. But for me, it was mostly cons because it made me feel like I was always just one of many potential options for each guy I was hooking up with." The sense that she was easily replaceable eventually produced enough anxiety that it affected her mental wellness.

She wanted a relationship in which she could feel safe, where she could connect authentically with another individual. Instead, she found herself stuck in a competitive space where Effortless Perfection was the standard, causing her to feel unattractive and disposable. Additionally, she hated that she didn't feel like she could explicitly project that she wanted more because there was a general belief that this would "send guys running."

Louise, who prefers not to mention her school, confirms, "If I could have asked for anything [from the guy I'd been consistently hooking up with as a first-year] it would have been 'Can we hold hands in public?' 'Can we get lunch in a space where people we know would see us?'" She learned the hard way that just because someone feels comfortable whispering sweet nothings in private does not mean exclusivity is in the cards.

Her way of responding to this dynamic was to "get drunk and hook up with other people because God forbid I make it look as though I genuinely like you and want to be with you because then I'm pathetic." Sociology and human sexuality professor at Occidental College Lisa Wade would call this move "performing meaninglessness" by going out of one's way to discount any emotional attachment they may be developing for the person(s) with whom they are involved.[4] What's one to do when the opposite—expressing meaning*ful*ness—is grounds for labeling someone, to use Louise's words, "crazy clingy"?

Like Anne and Louise, the majority of my interviewees had participated in hookup culture at one point or another. Some fully enjoyed it, some felt degraded by it, and some fell in middle of that spectrum. Surprisingly, what tied many of these women together was that their end goal was to eventually end up in a loving, committed relationship. *In many of their minds, the primary pathway to monogamy in college was to engage in hookup culture.*

While this may seem counterintuitive, Susana at Duke reasons, "This can be a totally healthy progression—if you like someone and you both have those desires, then I think it's natural to act upon it. The real issue is if someone in the pairing doesn't want to go there, but thinks they need to do so to keep the other person engaged." In her opinion, it is the one-sidedness and lack of natural desire that renders this kind of interaction a negative one, though she maintains that hooking up is too nuanced and the outcomes are too dependent to label engaging in it either a good or a bad thing.

This insight felt refreshing to me—here was a young woman who wasn't entirely for or against hookup culture. Rather, she had reflected on it and what she wanted from it and concluded the best way for her to navigate it, personally. Hookup culture wasn't something she fully accepted or rejected; it was a line she chose to walk.

Sammi at Duke also walked this line, though she had chosen her own specific trajectory after reevaluating her original reasons for hooking up: "As a freshman, I realized I was getting a lot of male attention and it definitely became a weird power trip, but simultaneously it made me a slave to obsessing over my weight and how I looked. It was all about getting that contact high of 'this guy wants me' and being able to pick and choose who 'got me.'" She believes it was ultimately unhealthy because the "weirdly addictive" self-esteem boosts she would experience each time she hooked up with a guy were something she could not find a way to feel on her own.

After much reflection, she came to the conclusion that, if she wanted to engage in hookup culture in a way she considered healthy, she needed to be much more in tune with her motivations. Furthermore, she needed to be conscious of her tendency to blur *what it means to be desired* (more physical) with *what it means to be valued* (more personal). Like Susana, Sammi found that reflecting on what she wanted and how to guide herself to those desired circumstances with more intention was an important part of making future interactions ultimately positive for her.

Overall, some undergrads benefit from and enjoy hookup culture, while others do not. It's not the difference in preference that's a problem; it's the way that conforming to hookup culture often gets presented as the only option if one wants to be seen as a fun, social person. Those who feel out of place in the hookup world often find themselves questioning: *Why is this so hard for me? Why do I care so much? Why can't I just casually hook up like everyone else? Why can't I disassociate myself from the need to be seen and valued before I feel comfortable hooking up? Why is this the opposite of effortless for me?*

When the expectation is that all college students be completely uninhibited about jumping into hookup culture, that view leaves anyone with reservations or complete discomfort feeling very isolated. Their sense of belonging often takes a hit. It's yet another way the Effortless Perfection Myth reinforces the notion that female undergrads are simply not enough the way they are.

Chapter 35

Hookup Culture's Exclusion of Minorities

SPEAKING OF BELONGING, consider how the heteronormativity[i] of hookup culture makes LGBTQ students feel. It's hard to feel a sense of belonging when the default system in place doesn't really recognize your existence. Even with its negatives, when hookup culture gets portrayed as one of the most quintessential elements of college (and a fundamental part of achieving Effortless Perfection), it can be devastating to feel so unincluded.

One student explains in a 2015 Me Too Monologue, "Every night out is the same—the frat, the bar, watching others hook up, the walk home alone. Each time I see a guy and a girl hook up, a piece inside of me dies because I don't even have that option. I can't just turn around and hook up with the nearest [person,] and seeing your tongue in [their] mouth flaunts that in my face."[1] Options are limited when only around eight percent of the U.S. adult population identifies as gay, lesbian, bisexual, or transgender. [2] (Though, that percentage appears to be increasing, as one in six members of Generation Z identify as LGBTQ according to a 2021 Gallup poll.)[3]

---

[i] Heteronormativity is the assumption that everyone involved in a given situation identifies as heterosexual, or "straight," when in reality heterosexuality is never a given. Heterosexuality is only one of the many possibilities of sexual expression. Gay, lesbian, bisexual, trans, queer, asexual, and gender-nonconforming individuals are almost always ignored when it comes to the setting of what are determined cultural "norms," especially in the case of hookup culture.

Plus, the dangers of expressing homosexual desires outside deemed "safe" spaces—like a gay bar or the university LGBTQ center—sometimes feel too great. When members of the LGBTQ community do decide to take the risk of engaging in a public display of affection, they are often hyperaware of the potential threats, insults, and jeers that may follow. (RTI International's report "*Violence and LGBTQ Communities: What Do We Know, and What Do We Need to Know?*" tracked 20 years of data through a combined sample of 73,000 LGBTQ youth and found bullying of this population has unfortunately not improved since the 1990s. LGBTQ students remain two to three times more likely than peers to be threatened or physically assaulted at school. Statistics of discrimination outside of educational facilities do not appear much better, unfortunately.)[4] It's impossible to predict how any one person in the crowd around them may react.

Louise recalls an evening when she was on a romantic date with her girlfriend, feeling so in love, all to have the mood ruined by a woman yelling at them on the street for holding hands and giving each other a peck on the cheek in front of her children. "When making the move to show your affection for another also has to come with such a strong association of fear, it messes with your natural instincts and blends two feelings together that really suck to have to feel at the same time," she attests.

Understandably, many members of the LGBTQ community are unwilling to come out at first. But that choice has its burdens, too. Louise explains that, before coming out, she constantly had to do a "big ol' dance" around pronoun usage in reference to the gender of her love interests. She was always bracing herself during conversations because she was worried about certain details of her life being revealed under the wrong circumstances.

"Putting so much additional thought and worry into your everyday behavior and communication is exhausting. It makes you want to limit your interactions sometimes because they just take so much mental and physical energy to get through," she explains. Before letting go of her secret, Louise often found herself feeling withdrawn, shrouded in the sensation that her ongoing way of being was somewhat "unnatural" because she was always putting on an act and presenting the world with a "lesser shade" of the person she really was. Who has time for Effortless Perfection when they're just trying to muster the energy to make it through their day?!

McKenzie at Duke knew that feeling all too well during the majority of her college experience. Trying to navigate her nonplatonic feelings for women while also dealing with fears about how her family and friends and the world in general would respond to her being lesbian was no easy task. She discusses the challenges she ran into as a female undergrad who did not fit into the heteronormative structure of hookup culture or the overall culture of Effortless Perfection at her school:

> *I came to [college] beyond confused about what I wanted. Initially, I decided that I should probably find a guy, given that that's what everyone else seemed to be doing. So I met like twenty of them by making out with them.... It was kind of fun in my [alcohol]-created haze.... Fun aside, I could never seem to find any footing at all. In January, my friends and I rushed, and landed in sororities that we loved, and still do to this day. But, while they thrived at their date functions and mixers, I felt empty. I felt like I didn't belong.... It took me two more years and a drunken make-out with a woman to realize exactly what I'd been missing.*

She admits with great frustration that this discovery did not immediately lead to "clarity and self-acceptance." She remained closeted—afraid of being put in a box and rejected. She felt she had nothing to gain by opening up and being vulnerable with others about this part of herself in an environment where Effortless Perfection was all about being the best possible version of "normal...whatever that means." There was nothing effortless about constantly questioning herself and her sexuality.

Many tears and bottles of wine later, McKenzie realized that "hiding felt worse than trusting [her] friends with the truth." So she took off her mask and stopped pretending and found herself pleasantly surprised at how accepting her close friends were. "Stories of spray-painted slurs and vandalized pride flags" no longer left her feeling completely alone because, now, she had a community she could rely on for support. She pushed past the damaging dominant narrative on campus and found an alternative narrative that suited her much better.

McKenzie's story elicits great hope because it shows just how powerful a personal transformation can be made in college when one pushes back against pressures to conform. Still, she faced a great number of challenges in getting to this better place. For instance, within the dominant narrative of campus hookup culture, a guy and a girl making out on the dance floor is nothing to bat an eye over. But if two women are doing it, it can be viewed as an invitation for harassment and fetishization.

She recalls kissing a girl off to the side of a party, only to have a guy walk up and ask: "Are you bi? Because I would be *down* with this." His interruption suggested that her make-out with this other woman was an overtly promiscuous display designed to draw male attention, when such an assumption would never be made if she were making out with a guy.

McKenzie also notes with frustration the way in which female-female relationships are often viewed as two women "experimenting" instead of something serious. She reflects, "There is this frustrating implication you are eventually going to flip back to men. Why is our interaction less legitimate based off the fact we both identify as women?" How completely invalidating!

Louise struggled with this same dilemma in her own way. For the first half of her college experience, she wrestled with the notion that she wasn't "gay enough to be gay" since she was still attracted to men.

"Bisexuality has little visibility and many people think of it as 'Oh, they are just going through a phase;' so for those of us who don't quite feel settled into knowing what we are yet, it can lead us to question: 'What if they are right?'" she notes.

As an underclassman, Louise wasn't just navigating the hookup world; she was simultaneously navigating her sexual orientation. She wanted to be able to claim "membership" in the LGBTQ community, thus gaining access to a group that could understand what she was going through, but there was still the part of her that feared her feelings weren't "fully cooked" enough.

After a while she realized, "If you think you like women then you probably do." She further jokes about this epiphany of hers: "There's no threshold you need to achieve—it's not like I need to have six crushes on women over the course of however many months and then I am a 'level-one lesbian' and I can tell people." Getting to this realization, however, was made much harder by the cultural climate around her. She had to push beyond stereotyping and ignorance to reach a place where she finally felt comfortable letting the world see her fullest self. Heteronormativity and the Effortless Perfection Myth be damned!

Even with the accompanying challenges of coming out, all the women I spoke to who identify as LGBTQ confirmed that speaking their truth was ultimately a positive experience. One described coming out as finally ridding herself of the "bowling ball" that had been growing inside her stomach all throughout high school and college.[5] From there, her comfortability with her sexuality only grew. "The transition from acceptance into pride feels like you are breathing air at full lung capacity for the first time," she revels. For her, openly defying the dominant narrative and freely living her own alternative narrative has been more than worth it in the long run.

Those who identify as LGBTQ aren't the only ones left out of the hook-up culture equation. Students of color, on average, hook up less than white students, too, which is often tied to fear of negative stereotyping and eroticization. Evette Dionne notes in an article for *Mic*: "Hook-up culture is racialized and full of classist assumptions of womanhood."[6]

Black women continue to be haunted by the hypersexual image of the jezebel[7], a stereotype that dates all the way back to when slavery was legal in the United States. The jezebel image was used to justify the horrific treatment Black women endured, including rape and other forms of sexual terrorization, by branding them as promiscuous and immoral. If they were portrayed as deviant nymphomaniacs ravenous for sex, then they couldn't possibly be raped because they were the ones doing the "luring." The stereotype is a whole new level of problematic.

Meanwhile, Latina women are often eroticized as "spicy" or "fiery" and Asian women are fetishized as submissive. These caricatures have left oppressive imprints on what behaviors women of color feel they can and cannot engage in if they do not want to be lumped into a demeaning burlesque.[8]

"Racism is at its most intense and ugly state in sexual relations," Maria believes. She laments that, after hooking up with guys outside her racial community, they tend to act in accordance with one of two opposite extremes. Either she is their dirty little secret who will never be more than a hookup because they don't think of her as someone to "bring home to meet the family" (for reasons that are subtly and not so subtly about race), or they "put that shit on blast and make sure everyone knows they 'smashed' a black girl."

Jessica somewhat similarly scoffs, "I've gotten a lot of 'I've never hooked up with an Indian girl before' or the more thinly veiled 'I've always wanted to hook up with someone *like you*.'" She finds that having to expect these kinds of loaded statements as a reality of participating in one of the most prominent aspects of the social scene to be infuriating. She attests, "It's exhausting to feel treated as a social experiment by a white guy who has never hooked up with a non-white girl." At the end of the day she just wants to feel desired "the same as anyone else" without being expected to fulfill some "exotic fantasy" or have "sexual magic tricks" in her back pocket.

The kind of attention these two women describe receiving is not so much an expression of desire as it is a form of fetishization. This is very problematic because, to have someone attracted solely to your cultural identity, as opposed to what you have to offer as an individual, is all too often rooted in oppressive expectations based on gross stereotyping. Fetishization is not an appreciation of a person of color's culture; it is a commodification of who and what they represent. It is usually the result of an extremely monolithic understanding of what it means to be a person of color in a way that is reductionist and dehumanizing.

In addition to hurtful biases from outside their racial community, women of color also have to deal with being policed by members of their own race due to respectability politics. As defined by my friend and brilliant academic Afftene Taylor, respectability politics are "the adherence to a set of choices, thought patterns, etcetera that are considered 'safe,' 'expected,' and/or 'understood to be normal or right' for a particular identity group." These moralistic principles are typically reinforced within more marginalized communities as a means of gaining greater social status.

Afftene asserts that Black women bear the brunt of respectability politics because "[we] are considered overtly sexual just due to the existence of our bodies—the pendulous breasts, the voluminous lips, the wide child-bearing hips. So much of it considered 'bad', 'dirty', 'sinful.'" Thus, they are expected to fight the stereotype that's been forced upon them by fitting themselves into a narrow definition of respectability that requires being "feminine presenting," "cisgender," and "a heterosexual virgin until marriage." The result is that large swaths of Black women are forced into "closets of shame," both by white people and by people from their own communities.

This keeps many from fully being themselves and engaging with the world in a way that is free and genuine. Afftene laments:

> *Just look at how we treat the few bold and brave Black women who decide to explore the fullness of themselves. They risk social condemnation, particularly in a community where togetherness means so much. If your own community turns on you or deems you as "unworthy," as a Black woman, who do you go to? Where do you run? What other group is gonna welcome you with open arms? You're a woman without a country.*

Talk about being in a bind. When the African American community already faces such a great deal of discrimination from the outside world, at least being respected *within* one's own community is critical. But what is one to do when the expectations of that community sometimes reinforce a form of internalized sexism?

Afftene recalls the way her mother preached this "respectability" to her as a child: "'Keep your drawers up and your dress down,' she would say." Her mother wouldn't even let her and her sister wear certain colored underwear because she feared it would "somehow trigger our sexuality and make us hos." Afftene may have laughed while recounting this, but her delivery also made clear a community-wide fear surrounding the developing bodies of young Black girls due to the accompanying hypersexualization and other forms of oppression that tend to exponentially mount as they mature.

This is not without reason. Consider this: the American Bar Association reports that convicted rapists of white women receive, on average, longer sentences than convicted rapists of women of color.[9]

Ultimately, this reveals a sexual hierarchy by which some women's bodies are deemed worthier of protection than others, which is beyond messed up. Whether caused by conscious or subconscious bias, the outcomes are very real and utterly devastating. Naturally, members of the African American community want to combat the very real danger such prejudices place upon them. The presence of respectability politics are complicated elements of this response.

Another woman of color with whom I spoke, Lily, brought up the moment when her mother admitted to her with shame that she had not been a virgin when she got married. Reflecting on it now, she wishes her mother had been more forthright: "If your ultimate goal was to make sure your children make healthy sexual decisions, don't get pregnant or come home with STDs, you didn't have to lie.... What about all the conversations we could have had?" Lily expresses her disappointment over the role respectability politics played in making those kinds of honest discussions harder to have: "I could have asked her, 'What it was like to have the feeling—I want to share my body with this particular person,' or 'How did you deal with it when a guy touched you in a particular way and it felt good?'" She feels robbed of that much yearned-for guidance.

Overall, the culture of shame that women of color experience regarding their bodies and the expression of their sexualities makes navigating the hookup/dating world even *more* difficult—as if it weren't already fraught enough! Many of those I interviewed argued that there were so many questions specific to them that had been left unanswered: *How am I supposed to take control of my sexuality and experience it in an empowering and liberating way without facing additional prejudice? What option is open to me, if any? And if conquering the hookup world is so central to achieving Effortless Perfection does that automatically kick me out of the running on the basis of my race? How on earth is any of this fair?*

Chapter 36

The Smokescreen of Hookup Culture

WITH THE OUTCOMES OF HOOKUP CULTURE equating to an overall net-negative for such a diverse range of individuals—for the majority of individuals, really—how is it that this system remains the apparent name of the game on college campuses? Why haven't those who are turned off by it, or even harmed by it, created some sort of alternate system? How does this culture persist?

Looking at today's media, the most hyped narrative regarding social life on college campuses is "sex as a sport, as a way of life, as a source of constant self-scrutiny and self-analysis."[1] A major component in competing to be Effortlessly Perfect is the social capital that comes from hooking up. It is the most visible social narrative. "Everyone is doing it," students tell themselves. But how true is that claim, really? Check it out:

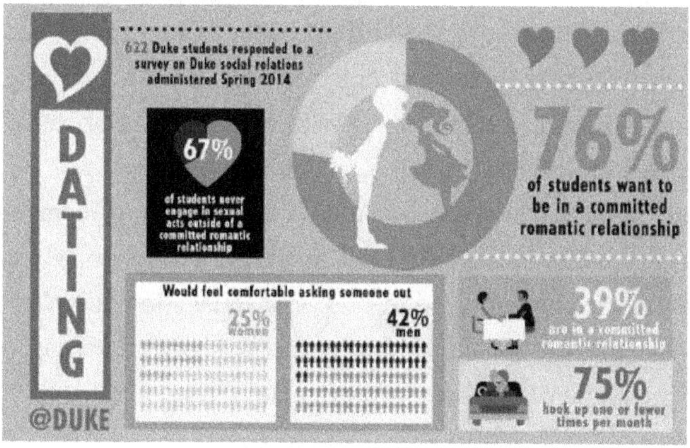

2

The first time I came across this graphic in my student newspaper, I was personally shocked. *How crazy,* I thought. *None of these statistics suggest a particularly strong presence of hookup culture on campus.* Sure, it was there, but it wasn't the only thing there. How could it be that word on the street was "no one dates here," when up to 39 percent of Duke students reported being in committed relationships and 67 percent claimed sexual acts outside of relationships were not something they wanted for themselves?

I looked into the study from which these statistics were pulled and was given irrefutable evidence that dating was actually happening at my college, and in much greater numbers than I ever would have guessed. According to the Duke Social Relationships Project, close to a quarter of students were dating someone locally, either on campus or nearby, with an additional 12 percent in long-distance relationships.[2] The study also showed that—of the two-thirds of Duke students not in committed romantic relationships—only a little over 50 percent had hooked up with someone in the previous six months. Furthermore, the 2014 Duke Inquiries on Social Relationships Study showed that three-fourths of respondents wanted to be in romantic relationships.[3]

A nationwide study with a data set comprised of survey responses from over 14,000 undergrads at 19 institutions of higher learning across the U.S. further reflected these trends. New York University sociology professor Paula England reported that, while 72 percent of students recounted participating in at least one hookup by their senior year, there were several important distinctions within this subset of individuals to consider. To start, physical activity during a hookup was not typically as "heavy" or "involved" as many assumed. Only one-third reported having engaged in actual intercourse in their most recent hookup, while another third reported having engaged in oral or manual stimulation of genitals, and the last third reported kissing without genital touching. Furthermore, of the 72 percent who had participated in hookup culture by their senior year, 40 percent had engaged three or fewer times, 40 percent had engaged four to nine times, and just 20 percent had engaged ten or more times. Thus, only 14 percent of the student population reported regularly hooking up. Lastly, 69 percent of heterosexual students reported having been in a college relationship of at least six months by their senior year, suggesting hookup culture had not entirely replaced traditional, committed relationships or kept them from forming.[5] So how exactly did hooking up come to dominate the conversation, or even define it?

This misperception is the result of the same issue we have been discussing in parallel with the Effortless Perfection Myth all along—that the dominant narrative all too often overshadows the *full* narrative. In the case of hookup culture, the majority of undergrads privately reject the perceived norm, while incorrectly assuming most others accept it.

In her book *The End of Sex,* Donna Freitas writes, "Most students are able to readily define how hookups function as social capital on campus—and their definitions are fairly uniform.... However, many students report what they believe the practice entails *according to everyone else,* as if they did not participate in the practice themselves."[6] If those being influenced by the perceived norm had a way of seeing that their reading of the situation is misguided, they would be able to self-correct, but because of fears they will be ostracized for not participating, they remain silent so as not to draw attention to themselves.

Thus, it would appear hookup culture is more a smokescreen than anything else. Yet somehow that smoke has managed to find its way under the cracks of our doors, filling our dorm rooms with a smoldering scent that leads us to believe any potential for real dating on our respective campuses has gone up in flames. Collegiate women act accordingly, assuming this is "just the way things are," despite the fact that this perceived norm does not accurately reflect reality.

Collegiate guys act accordingly, too. Though men are typically assumed to be the main benefactors (perhaps even perpetrators) of hookup culture, many feel just as dissatisfied by the norms of hookup culture as women do. Dr. Glass notes:

> *It is not uncommon to encounter young men seeking counseling for something that reflects anxiety, depression, or simply the loneliness and fears of whether they are living well. Also not uncommon is the disclosure that their social circles, often those in fraternities, are linked to these struggles in that these young men are disconnected from their more genuine selves looking for real and intimate connections...they describe wishing for a deeper connection but are urged, teased, or applauded into conforming to a hookup culture that prohibits anything that resembles connection or commitment to an actual relationship.*[7]

Such social pressures call upon young men to showcase their dominance, to make a demonstration of their social control via displays of heavy drinking, rowdiness, and "pulling" enough girls to meet the "hookup quota." While some may revel in and feel completely at ease with this version of "guy" culture, many do not. They just don't feel comfortable admitting that out loud, so most women aren't able to realize that these kinds of men are out there, too. Which is unfortunate, because our lives would be a lot easier if they would let themselves be known!

Overall, hooking up is not some necessary hump to get over before a relationship begins. We need to communicate the following message, loud and clear: *If hooking up is not what you want, it's okay to ask for what you really desire. If only parts of it are for you, it's okay to communicate that, too. You may be surprised by how many others feel the same. Don't be fooled by the smokescreen.*

Section VI

Settling into Our True Identities

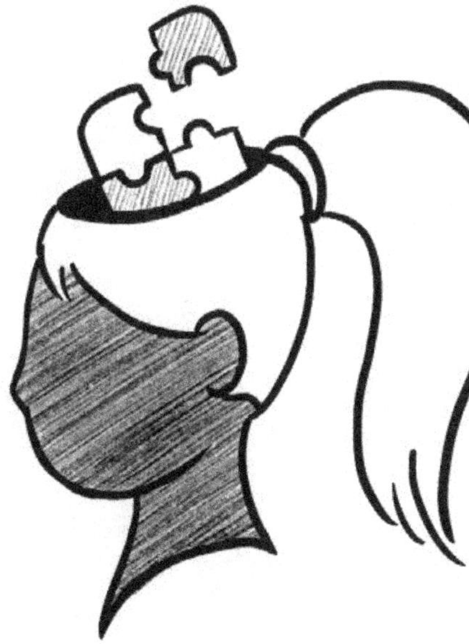

Chapter 37

Trading Our Values for a Sense of Belonging

SELF-ESTEEM, confidence, assertiveness, body image, hookup culture—there are an overwhelming number of issues to navigate in college. All of them play a role in how undergraduate women feel about ourselves and the choices we make, which ultimately determines the identities we develop.

Identity is a complicated issue. Are we the labels we place upon ourselves, or the labels others place upon us? Or maybe we are only the labels that we *allow* others to place upon us? And what if labels don't really matter at all?

I saved the topic of identity for the last section of this book because I believe it to be at the heart of a fulfilling college and life experience. With a strong sense of identity often comes a strong sense of purpose, so the further we develop our own sense of who we are and what we want out of life, the more the extemporaneous issues lose their power to distract and hinder us. Gradually, it becomes easier to determine what matters and what doesn't, commit our focus to the things that do, and let the rest fade into the background.

Effortless Perfection confuses the hell out of that process because it dictates what our identity should be and what we should care about, leaving little room for anything else. It is a "self-erasing identity" that promises to help us stand out and reach our fullest potential, but really just has us chasing the status quo like a dog chasing a squirrel.[1]

So how does one actually go about developing a strong identity instead of pursuing the empty image of Effortless Perfection? First, we need to understand how identity operates. Identity is comprised of two principles:

- The need to feel unique, with one's own sense of personal agency and value
- The need to feel a sense of belonging within a community that shares similarities with us

To stand out, but fit in. To be different, but the same. The paradox this inserts into our lives can be hard to navigate.

Dr. Stephen Hinshaw, a psychology expert specializing in adolescent development, observes that this interplay can come across as instructions: *"Be yourself, but not too much. Be proud of you are, but only so long as how you look, speak, and think is appealing to others. Be one-of-a-kind, but in the right way, not the wrong way."*[2] However, these two principles are not contradictory so much as they are in competition. A solid sense of identity boils down to finding proper balance between the two.

Still, this is easier said than done. It goes without saying that we, as human beings, are social creatures. We are wired to pursue connection with others. We crave to feel seen and heard by our peers. Study after study has shown that a sense of belonging is critical to one's well-being.[3] In fact, fMRI studies reveal that the same areas of the brain light up when we experience rejection as when we experience physical pain. Social exclusion piggybacks on those same neural pathways.[4]

In novel situations where individuals are new to a community and just beginning to create support systems of friends and acquaintances, they are typically more willing to sacrifice agency and set certain values aside because not feeling like there is a place one fits in and belongs can be really painful. Particularly as undergrads first arrive at college, a sense of desperation sometimes kicks in when we are not immediately able to recreate the kinds of support groups we had back home. That sense of desperation causes many of us to put all our efforts into the "belonging" aspect of our identity, while forgetting to attend to the "individuality" aspect of our identity.

I will never forget the feeling of ripping open my letter on Bid Day to reveal the emblem of the sorority for which I had been hoping. My stomach was doing backflips. Months later it was still doing flips, but for an entirely different reason.

By this point my freshman year, I'd spent countless hours going to mixers and date functions with the primary goal of becoming closer with my pledge class. But these events continued to feel like a continuous series of pop quizzes meant to test my social capabilities for the level of entertainment I could provide—as if every interaction was a test drive to see if I was worth getting to know.

I was exhausted from the charade. I remember thinking to myself, *This is not fine. I am not okay. It is truly incredible how inferior I can allow myself to feel. What authority did they have to make me feel this way?*

I wanted to just disconnect the wires in my brain that made me care so much about what everyone else thought of me. But, at the same time, I so badly hoped to be understood by each and every one of them. I wanted them to see the ability I possessed within me to be a loyal friend, to understand the trueness of my intentions. I wanted them to care about me, or at least to *like* me. My thought process circled the same question over and over again: *What am I doing wrong?*

There are still pictures on Facebook of the nights when I was "lucky" enough to be invited along. I look so happy. It's the type of picture I could show to my daughter twenty years from now: "Mommy with her sorority sistaaahs!" All of us holding the quintessential red cups in some frat house with that black miniskirt I used to rock. We are freeze-framed in a moment that screams youth and "the best days of our lives."

But I remember what that night was really like. The house was pretty empty when we arrived, so we spent the majority of our time taking picture after picture. All those laughing snapshots are posed. And the girl with her arm around me, there, kept purposely cutting me out of the tight dance circle later that night.

In these pictures, it looks like I've achieved Effortless Perfection. It looks like I belong. But I know that if I had truly belonged, I wouldn't have felt so alone. I wouldn't have felt the need to evaluate every word I said or to think about what every person's body posture meant or to subconsciously strategize how to win people's favor.

I'd believed that, if I could just make myself into who I thought they wanted me to be, I would be awarded that sense of belonging I so craved from the social group that had theoretically hand-chosen me to be one of them. Instead, I watched myself shrink and conform into a shell of my former self.

I just didn't get what was expected of me and I felt like I could not succeed in meeting my own expectations if I did not have a clear understanding of how I was to meet the expectations of others. I'd created a warped reality wherein I could not fully love myself unless I was loved by everyone else.

Clearly this was an unrealistic expectation, an impossible standard of never butchering a first impression while playing by everyone else's unwritten, unspoken rules. And yet here I was trying to prove to everybody I met that I was witty and charming and fully worthy of their attention, both people who shared my values and those who did not. So even if she was looking over my shoulder as we spoke for someone more popular than me to talk to or he was probably just prowling for that night's hookup, I subconsciously allowed myself to feel disappointed, maybe even ashamed, that they didn't seem to place value on me.

Multiple interviewees expressed to me that they had similar experiences in their college social scenes. In our efforts to make inroads with our new peers, we became too quick to jump onto the bandwagon of the dominant narrative without checking to make sure the direction that wagon was headed was where we really wanted to be going. In doing so, not only did we end up compromising personal agency and unique individuality, but we often ended up compromising some of our personal values, too. In short, *we traded our values for a chance to fit in.*

Aurora at Vanderbilt admits that, as an underclassman, she dumbed herself down, played the role of the "cool, chill girl," and developed a hyperawareness of her tendency to speak loudly. She found herself staying at parties where she wasn't enjoying herself long into the evening because it was the place to be seen that night. Her typically bright and colorful wardrobe slowly became entirely black to match the NYC vibes her sorority was theoretically supposed to be emulating.

She had gone through rush thinking, "If they don't like me as I am, then I don't belong there," but once she was a member she found herself stuck in an unforeseen snafu. "I was already in.... but didn't feel like I was actually in. I still had to work to be included and prove I could hang," she explains. She attributes the sense of belonging she finally established in college to finding a group of people—some inside her sorority, but mostly outside—that she felt comfortable being her fullest self around.

Aurora's remarks remind me of a secret one of my peers revealed in a low whisper during a diversity immersion retreat we attended together. As a woman of color belonging to a majority-white sorority, she felt a "messed-up need" to always be at the "top of her game" to be the "'fun' token Asian girl." She felt this to the point where, if she did not think she could live up to this role 100 percent on a given night, she would just stay in. The demand for her to look and present herself in a very specific, exaggerated manner was exhausting and only allowed her to present one facet of her identity to the world. Yet she couldn't push away the feeling that this was required of her if she wanted to maintain a sense of belonging.

Not feeling fully accepted by one's community or social environment can evoke urgent, anxious responses. It is natural to react by looking for patterns, or some sort of key to reveal to us: *This is what you need to do and who you need to be to be accepted here.* Unfortunately, this is when the zeitgeist of Effortless Perfection finds its ideal moment to strike. We put our trust in that zeitgeist and work tirelessly, in vain, to meet its demands.

That is, until we learn the difference between truly belonging and just fitting in. In the words of Brené Brown: "Belonging is being somewhere you want to be, and they want you. Fitting in is being somewhere you really want to be, but they don't care one way or the other."[5] There is a major difference between being accepted for who we are versus being allowed to tag along because of how closely we can make ourselves resemble the status quo. Those dedicated to chasing Effortless Perfection will never achieve a real sense of self-actualization, of meeting both aspects of their identity needs because they will forever be stuck in the pattern of trading the second for the first.

The trick is to find a group (or groups) that recognize and accept all the ways in which you are different in addition to your shared similarities. My sorority may not have been that place, but my campus had plenty of other options; I just needed to find them. While on the hunt, there were moments I felt like I was floating out to space, but when I did finally find the circles that celebrated and pursued the same kinds of things I celebrated and pursued, while also appreciating my unique personality traits, I was home. I no longer felt like an ugly stepsister trying to force my foot into a shoe that did not fit. The sense that I had to shove down or hold back major parts of who I was in order to achieve status within the group was nowhere to be found. I was free to meet all my identity needs and be all of myself.

Chapter 38

Pursuing an Image Versus Developing an Identity

THE SIMPLEST WAY to shift out of Effortless Perfection's never-ending cycle of please, appease, and perform is to recognize the difference between pursuing an image versus developing an identity.

An image is something one must constantly strive for, a process that transforms us from human beings into "human doings." We fall into patterns of "I will be happy when I ________ (get into med school, reach this weight, catch so-and-so's attention)," which try to create proof that we are winning whatever it is we are supposed to be winning. We create a system by which we are attempting to build a sense of self out of grade-point average, Instagram likes, and other forms of academic and social capital.

In contrast, an identity is something we take on when we recognize that we are enough as we are now. It is something we are, simply by being and living in the moment—no proof or validation necessary because it doesn't have to measure up to standards defined by anybody other than ourselves.

The biggest difference between the two is that an identity is permanent, while an image can only be achieved in brief moments. We reach it and embody it, but then the moment shifts or the image alters and we fall back into hot pursuit. It's exhausting, like running on a treadmill that only goes faster.

In college, I was on this treadmill at a dead sprint until I asked myself: *Why does it matter how fast I can run if I'm not actually making ground?* I realized that I needed to make a change, but failing to fit this image of Effortless Perfection felt like a loss of the only thing I knew how to be, the only self I knew how to pursue. I wasn't ready to give up control.

If only I'd known that I feared this lack of "control" because I'd convinced myself that breaking from my pursuit of perfection would mean certain chaos, when in fact it meant freedom. Freedom to ask myself more important questions than "What will everyone think?" but rather "What makes me, me?" It was this shift from pursuing an image to developing an identity that allowed me to switch my internal dialogue from "Who am I *supposed* to be?" to "Who do I *want* to be?"

Now, I'll be the first to admit, there will always be parts of me that want to press the speed button up a bit on the treadmill and willingly chase that image of perfection. This can be so tempting, for it seems so promising. But I've come to understand that we have somewhat of a choice in selecting the criteria by which we determine our own self-worth, so why not push toward something that's more inclined to make us feel good about ourselves?

The desire to curate and to project an image of perfection is present nowhere more than it is on social media. Riley at Vanderbilt knows all too well what it means to struggle to live up to a particular image, particularly on Instagram and Snapchat. "Sometimes I take a pic and spend hours honing which exact filter I want to use, how to crop it.... Thinking about what carefully crafted caption would be most enticing for others to read," she notes. She also mentions the "widespread knowledge" that, in order to get the most likes, posts should be uploaded in the middle of the day or right before people go to bed when they are most likely to be scrolling.

Visibility of content is an important component of a well-managed social media account—our generation's most obvious form of personal branding. While admitting to being very much wrapped up in all of this, Riley also recognizes that social media is about perpetuating an image of oneself that does not usually delve beneath the surface. She has mixed feelings about what this means.

Social media is not inherently bad; how we use it is what matters. *Ultimately, it boils down to whether we are using it to connect or to compete and compare.* We need to ask ourselves: Am I using these platforms to make a statement about what I think and care about? Am I connecting with issues or media campaigns that are bigger than myself?[1]

Or am I using these platforms to determine where I "stand" in comparison to my peers? Am I lurking[2]—passively viewing other's posts while sharing nothing myself—to catch a glimpse of what others are up to, to see if any of my friends made plans without me or if there are parties going on that I wasn't invited to? Am I interpreting "likes" and "followers" as an actual set of metrics for my social success?

Researchers call this second set of behaviors "social comparison and feedback seeking," noting it is strongly associated with depressive symptoms. In her 2015 *New York Times* article "Suicide on Campus and the Pressure of Perfection," Julie Scelfo theorizes that, for undergrads, "[t]he existential question 'Why am I here?' is usually followed by the equally confounding 'How am I doing?'"[3] In our quest to determine our standing, we use the tools of comparison available to us, tools that have exponentially multiplied in number and scope since the advent of social media outlets like Facebook, Instagram, Snapchat, TikTok, and the like.

This issue was brought to the forefront of national attention by Kate Fagan's ESPNW article "Split Image." Her piece drew a spotlight to the tragic death of Madison Holleran, a freshman track star at UPenn who appeared to have the "picture perfect" life, yet died by suicide early her second semester.[4, i(5, 6)]Just an hour before jumping from the top of a parking garage, Madison uploaded a fairy-tale-esque image of holiday lights twinkling from the trees in Rittenhouse Square right off campus. Among the other photos on her Instagram account of her playing sports, hanging with friends, and enjoying the company of family, this picture seemed like yet another indicator of a perfectly happy eighteen-year-old who was well adjusted to her new college life. The Effortlessly Perfect images she posted masked the reality that she had been depressed for several months.

Fagan writes of Madison: "She seemed acutely aware that the life she was curating online was distinctly different from the one she was actually living. Yet she could not apply that same logic when she looked at the projected lives of others."[7] Day in and day out, Madison was absorbing the images posted by peers she barely knew—images no different from the ones she was posting—*wondering why her life didn't feel the way everybody else's looked.* As she wandered through heavily filtered renditions of others' mini-feeds, she traversed her own unedited life wondering where she had gone wrong.

Of course, there was more to blame than social media; the state of her mental health obviously contributed greatly to her interpretation of the messages she was receiving. Still, in today's world, where our digital lives are so closely interwoven with both our public and private selves, it can be hard to tell what is real and what is not. Throw in the added dynamics of the drive to present or "brand" oneself in the most Effortlessly Perfect way, as well as the dependence on outside validation that social media fosters, and it is hard to differentiate between the image you are projecting and the actual identity you are developing.

---

i Suicide is the second-leading cause of death among fifteen- to twenty-four-year-olds (right after unintended motor vehicle accidents). Eighteen- to twenty-five-year-olds are more likely to experience suicidal thoughts than any other age group and attempt suicide at significantly higher rates, though their attempts are less likely to be fatal when compared to attempts by older age groups.

Social media has been a major component in bolstering the effects of the Effortless Perfection Myth that so easily brings us to question: *Why am I the only person who seems to be struggling?* In reality, all of us have issues with which we grapple. We just don't tend to post them, or talk about them, or really even acknowledge them in public forums.

Social media can act as a chorus of critics or a salient support group, depending on who we let in. It helps to be more intentional and selective about whom we follow. Accounts that do nothing but make us feel the need to be someone else should be unfollowed. Accounts that touch on deeper issues and embrace being authentically vulnerable should be sought out. It may seem odd to consider the choices we make on social media as part of our self-care routine, but they absolutely are. The content we post and follow plays a role in determining how well we prioritize the mindset of identity over image, and we must choose the former if we wish to overcome the mental health crisis being spurred by the Myth.

Chapter 39

The Link Between Effortless Perfection and Mental Health

AT A TIME IN OUR LIVES when so much is changing, college can be an especially vulnerable mental health period for many of us. It certainly was for me. As someone who had been identified as a sort of "golden girl" at her high school via various awards and lofty expectations, I'd gone off to college fully believing I was on the ultimate path to success. So a couple of years in, when I found myself curled up on a couch in a psychologist's office with my head cradled in my father's lap, overcome with a hopeless, drowning feeling I'd just been told was called depression, I felt betrayed by the universe.

On the way out the door after the meeting, I sniffled, "Why did this happen to me, Dad? This wasn't supposed to happen to me."

"This isn't supposed to happen to anyone, darlin'. What makes you so special?" he responded, looking at me with the most loving but honest eyes.

In that moment, I was forced to realize that my ability to conform to Effortless Perfection in no way entitled me to a life without struggle. I was struck by the disparity between what I'd figured I was allowed to expect and what had actually ended up happening. I couldn't help but feel disillusioned: *I gave it everything I had and it still wasn't enough. What was there left to do?*

I had believed that Effortless Perfection would serve as my suit of armor. Because the Myth had called for so much of my energy and life force to be directed toward its pursuit, I assumed things would work out for me if I followed its doctrine as painstakingly close as possible. After all, why would anyone chase something that demands so much from us for anything less?

But the Myth's promise was empty. The thing I had though would make me feel safe, my perfectionist drive, actually led me straight off the deep end.

Unfortunately, anxiety and depression are not abnormal college experiences. According to the 2013 National College Health Assessment, which examined data from 125,000 students at more than 150 institutions of higher learning, "About one-third of U.S. college students had difficulty functioning in the last twelve months due to depression, and almost half said they felt overwhelming anxiety in the last year."[1] Furthermore, the National Alliance on Mental Illness found that, while only 7 percent of parents report that their children are experiencing mental health issues in college, a full 50 percent of college students rate their mental health as below average or poor.[2]

If that weren't enough, depression has also been found to disproportionately affect women. Our likelihood of experiencing a depressive episode is the same as our male peers in childhood, but once early adolescence hits that rate steadily rises. By late adolescence, we are twice as likely as our male counterparts to experience depression—a trend that continues throughout adulthood.[3] A nineteen-year-old female has a one in five chance of already having experienced a depressive episode, and an even higher likelihood of having encountered minor or mild symptoms of depression.[4] How as a society have we reached such extremes?! From where does all of this stem?

The probability one will experience depression ultimately boils down to two things—genes and environmental triggers. Depression is a biochemical condition and, depending on our genes, some of us are more prone based on our brain chemistry. However, whether or not certain elements of those genes express themselves depends on external factors such as stress and trauma, which "activate" them.[5] For instance, an individual who has inherited a susceptibility to "brain chemistry imbalance" may feel stress and tragedy more deeply than an individual without that susceptibility would. As more negative life experiences occur, their vulnerability to mental health struggles increases at an exponential rate.[6]

Environments demanding Effortless Perfection are no doubt full of these activator-type experiences. In a column for *Inside Higher Ed*, Dr. Gary Glass emphasizes the level of anxiety created when operating on competitive campuses where so many seem to be "pursuing a vaguely defined success, fueled by a perpetual fear of failure."[7] In fact, I'm not sure if our generation recognizes just how much it is motivated by anxiety. If I think back, the grades I worked painstakingly hard to achieve in high school and college were not entirely the result of a love of learning. My frame of mind was not "If I do well, good things will happen," so much as "I have to do this because if I fail the outcomes will be dire."

This was true even more so for Aurora at Vanderbilt. As the first person in her family to go to college, she suffered from "deep imposter syndrome" that resulted in runaway anxiety and other mental health concerns. Without parents who knew how to guide her through the experience, she made it her mission to take everything head-on. She needed to do it all, and do it all very, very well. But there were consequences to the pressure she placed upon herself to achieve.

She details, "In middle school, I would throw up. In high school, I would break out in hives. In college, I got bad mouth ulcers and even had to be hospitalized for exhaustion one time. It was this anxiety that drove me—a fear of falling behind." She looked around at her Vanderbilt peers and noted the internships they were landing, where they were from, how affluent they seemed to be. Those things became her benchmark for what success looked like. She never considered how far she'd already come, only how far she had left to go.

Effortless Perfection on college campuses has created the "mass delusion" that there is one singular path one must follow in order to achieve a successful life.[8] The constant worry and fear about qualifying as this very specific kind of "successful" makes those on the Effortless Perfection pilgrimage highly susceptible to mental health issues like burnout and depression because one step off the path feels like disaster.

In a famous sermon by Maurice Boyd, an acclaimed New York minister, a parallel is drawn between perfection and anguish. He preaches of a world-renowned glassworks producer dating back to the 1700s: "At Waterford Crystal, each piece of crystal is meticulously inspected, held up to the light, each surface appraised for the slightest crack or deformity. If any is spotted, the piece is immediately shattered…for a defect nearly invisible to the human eye. Notice how close perfection is to despair."[9] When the flip side of perfection is obliteration, how could one not feel like everything they are is constantly at stake?

We need to see our pursuit of Effortless Perfection for what it is—a publicly applauded form of self-abuse.

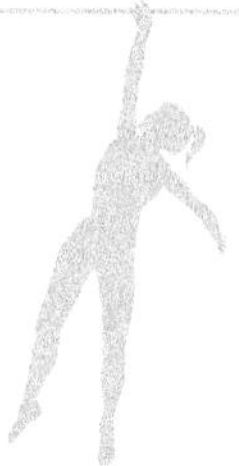

Chapter 40

Struggling with an "Unearned" Diagnosis

ANYONE WHO HAS EVER STRUGGLED with their mental health knows how incredibly difficult it can be to figure out what is happening inside of your head, let alone explain it to those around you. Mental health conditions are only made worse by the associated stigmas that all too often point a finger right back at the individual struggling.

Until I experienced my depressive episode, I had always believed happiness was somewhat of a choice. I thought it was about connecting to the bigger picture and resetting one's frame of mind. Suddenly, I was incapable of doing anything close to that and it felt like an utter and complete moral failing.

A peer of mine expressed her frustration over this same feeling via a brave Facebook post: "If there's one thing I've learnt, it's that no one should be ashamed of being sick. There is no other disease I know where the onus is put on the person suffering to 'cure themselves'—it makes no sense. I have spent too much time fluctuating from trying to see a false beauty in my depression to pretending it does not exist—it is exhausting and a waste of energy."[1] She further explains how the self-blame she initially floundered beneath only further "crippled" her desire to reach out for help. It made her believe that if she was "weak enough to succumb to depression" then she "deserved all its byproducts,"[2] which just goes to show how hazardous the pressure to "snap out of it" can be.

As I interviewed more and more women on Effortless Perfection and its related issues, I noticed a perplexing trend. *Not only do we seem to be competing for who is the best, but we seem to also be competing for who has it the worst (while still managing to stay on track)*. Bizarre as this may sound, many of those with whom I spoke brought up feeling like they "had not earned" their various mental health struggles because whatever they were going through wasn't "bad or extreme enough" for them to be feeling the way they were feeling.

Take this quote by my peer Lucy, which appeared in a 2014 "Humans of Duke" photo project:

> *A lot of times I feel like I'm not allowed to complain, to be upset, or stressed, because whatever's on my plate isn't…horrible enough. Most of my freshman year, I was depressed and I had been for a while. I never went to anybody because I thought I was just being shallow. There are people in way worse situations than I am. Nothing has really happened to me and I didn't think I "deserved" to be depressed. Isn't that silly? But I think it might be a common thing.*

The knowledge that other people had gotten themselves equally as far as she had, from much harder circumstances, made Lucy feel like she did not "deserve" a diagnosis.

I noticed the women of color and children of immigrants that I interviewed especially felt this way. Maria explained that, when she finally gathered the courage to tell her parents she thought she might be clinically depressed her sophomore year, they wrote depression off as "a white people issue" and "a rich people issue." Her parents had come to the United States as refugees and given everything they had to set their children up for better lives. Here she was attending college, with access to resources beyond their wildest dreams, and she was depressed? It did not add up to them. They felt uncomfortable calling it what it was. She explains:

> *I know this is a generalization, but I've noticed while living here that white [Americans] like to label and categorize things.... My parents don't feel comfortable doing the same because once you name "it," that's when it gains its power. That's when you engage with the idea that there might be something wrong with you or me or us. So, it's like, "If you call what you have depression, then what are you going to call the scary thoughts I have in* my *head? How are you selfish enough to say you are going through this? Don't you know what* I've *been through?"*

Claiming the title of "depressed" when others she knew had been through "so much more" made her feel guilty. She felt she did not deserve the "privilege of being able to label [her] pain," when doing so had been denied to so many others before her.

She struggled as the first generation of her family to be equipped with the language to say, "What I'm feeling right now is depression," or "What I'm feeling right now is anxiety." While she found this new vocabulary necessary for effectively describing her emotional struggles, she did not feel like it was welcome conversation in her community.

A 2014 study on African Americans' attitudes toward mental illness found that, while stigmas are decreasing within this community, older generations are still inclined to believe mental illness is "a sign of weakness and lack of inner strength."[3] This can be the case in other minority racial groups, as well. The 2017 California Well-Being Survey found that Asian Americans in the state reported higher levels of self-stigma than Caucasians in regard to mental illness. Latinos interviewed in English also reported higher levels of self-stigma, while Latinos interviewed in Spanish reported lower levels of stigma, though they were also the least likely of all racial and ethnic groups to have used mental health services.[4]

No wonder so many of the women I interviewed who had experienced mental health struggles described a strong sense of guilt about reaching out to others. They feared "wasting others' time," "making loved ones upset," and "piling on unnecessary baggage their friends and family didn't need." They didn't want to be a burden. Some also mentioned fear of being judged according to the stereotype of Millennials and Gen-Zers as generations obsessed with themselves and their own satisfaction without regard for ideals like responsibility and the greater good.

Stigmas surrounding mental health fail to recognize that environmental factors are only part of the equation. As previously stated, depression is a biochemical condition and, depending on the genes that have been passed down, some of us are more prone to depression based on brain chemistry. The comparison of "this person experienced this and was fine, so why can't I power through and be fine, too," is an unfair judgment of mental toughness and coping efforts.

Someone who has inherited a greater susceptibility to stress, anxiety, and depression may feel trauma and tragedy more intensely than an individual without that susceptibility would. "You don't need to have this horrible traumatic experience to hurt," Jane says. "It doesn't have to be suicide to be depression. It does not have to be rape to be sexual assault. Hurt is hurt. Pain is pain. It's not a contest."

Fear that our pain is not valid urges us to keep it locked inside instead of seeking the resources and group commiseration we need most, which is a problem because we can't do our best to help each other heal if none of us feel worthy of accepting the help and relief we each have to offer one another! We need to learn to say to ourselves: Yes, I *do* deserve the validation of knowing this issue is bigger than just me. This issue *is* something I deserve help fighting.

Chapter 41

Manufacturing Certainty

PURSUING EFFORTLESS PERFECTION and experiencing mental health setbacks are highly correlated events, in large part due to their relationship with control. As previously discussed, Effortless Perfection is not some petty, superficial issue based on upholding flawless appearances. For many of today's young women in college, pursuit of Effortless Perfection is an all-encompassing coping mechanism seeking to erase uncertainty from one's life. It is based on a false promise: *If I can make myself look perfect then I can expect my life to feel perfect, too.*

Brooke attests that for much of college her mindset was: "If something is perfect then it is in a 'complete state' and it can't be questioned. It has no weaknesses." Thus, her approach to the world around her was to limit the variability of things like romantic relationships, popularity, and academic success by approaching them as facets of her life to be mastered and maintained.

She had believed, "If I'm amazing at everything in every area of life, I can't get hurt because being perfect means nothing has to change so nobody will ever complain about me or reject me or pick fights with me. I will possibly even reach a form of enlightenment." In some ways this approach worked well for her. She had been the valedictorian of her high school. She had given modeling a shot in college and been successful.

However, this theory of hers unraveled as she was forced to reckon with the reality that this mindset ignored all the variables outside of her control. Take relationships, for example. Even if she worked very hard on her end of her relationships with friends or significant others, she was only half the equation. "When there is a whole other person added to the mix, they have the right to disagree, to change their mind, to go a different direction," she points out.

If our approach to life does not acknowledge that there will always be things out of our control, it's going to lead us down an infuriating path. *We cannot create expectation based upon unavailable certainty.* All that this does is throw us down the rabbit hole of endlessly extrapolating, "Okay, but what *if if if...*"

Meanwhile, we have no control over the ifs. Believing we do means that, when the expectations we've made based upon unavailable certainty do not come to fruition, the whole system upon which we have set our sense of security is shaken and it's a quick ride to desperation and hopelessness. We cannot out-think and out-worry the difficulties awaiting us in the future. Things simply do not work that way.

When I find myself on the *if if if* train, already thinking a hundred dominoes down the road about all the bad things that could happen that are out of my control, I like to remind myself that, if I flip the script, there is actually a positive way to employ this mode of thinking. Instead, I try to ask myself questions like: "What if everything works out?" "What if there is an opportunity I'm destined for that is better than what I've imagined for myself?"

Furthermore, I consider one of my favorite Mark Twain quotes: "I've lived through some terrible things in my life, some of which actually happened." What this quote means to me is that, when we allow stress and anxiety over the future to seep so strongly into the present moment, we suffer intensely from things that haven't and may not ever happen. We experience them as if they were occurring right at this very moment, thus loading an emotional burden onto our shoulders that we may not need to carry at all, ever. We do this all in the name of outwitting uncertainty—an impossible task that will never actually give us the security we crave—just high blood pressure!

In Eve Ensler's book *Insecure at Last*, she raises the point that obsession with security tends to cause individuals and societies to overestimate the level of danger present to them at any given moment. The Myth is no different; it leads us to feel like we're constantly one step away from falling off the precipice of perfection, straight into disaster. Such a mindset can be incredibly limiting to our development and life fulfillment. Ensler writes:

> *When security is paramount, you can't travel very far or venture too far outside a certain circle. You can't allow too many conflicting ideas in your mind at one time, as they may confuse or challenge you. You can't open yourself to new experiences, new people, and new ways of doing things.*
>
> *...All this striving for security has in fact made you much more insecure. Because now you have to watch out all the time....You have places you cannot go, thoughts you cannot think, worlds you can no longer inhabit. You spend your days fighting things off, defending your territory, and becoming more entrenched in your narrow thinking. Your days become devoted to protecting yourself. This becomes your mission. This becomes all you do."*[1]

She explains that when the mission is security before all else, we adapt ways of thinking that "freeze" and "numb" us in order to protect us from change or doubt. We think our rigid, obsessive behavior is keeping us safe, but it is really just shutting down our minds and our logic. In reality, we are not a single drop safer.

Sure, there is comfort in habit and familiarity, but sometimes we cling to what we instinctively know—the way Brooke clung to her perfectionism, and I clung to my eating disorder—and it ends up hurting us far more than helping us. The promise of certainty and security imbedded in these behaviors is a lie. The illusion it creates, ironically, just reduces and imprisons us.

The false protections Effortless Perfection offers us are heavy to lug around. They weigh us down because, as Ensler says, "Whatever secretly terrifies [us] ultimately controls [us]—determines how [we] feel, think, and behave."[2] In turn, she poses this question: What would happen if we reenvisioned our end goals and considered what life might look like "if security were not the point of our existence?"[3] What if we forfeited the false belief that we can control the outcomes of our lives by fearing and clinging and performing until we have no energy left to feel our vulnerability? What if we stopped the pointless charade of trying to make the uncertain certain and instead shifted the focus of that energy to love, curiosity, and exploration?

I'll be the first to admit, it makes sense to want to feel like the luxuries of life we experience are rewards for good behavior—that we have earned the things in our lives that are good by being good. We want fairness. We want to speak in a language of entitlements and calculate according to the careful math of deserving. In such a world, "nothing clung to could ever slip away" and there would be "no such thing as undeserved pain," to quote the words of Dr. Kate Bowler, author of *Everything Happens for a Reason and Other Lies I've Loved.*[4]

In reality, the hard truth is that being a "good"—let alone perfect—person does not tie you any tighter to the promise of a good life than other people. I was forced to confront this after witnessing the tragic death of a friend while abroad in college. She was a big ball of joy, a driven student committed to public service, and a deeply loved daughter and friend. And then she was gone. I wanted a reason. I wanted the certainty and sense of control such a reason might give me. But there wasn't one.

Digging for a greater reason in the name of certainty carried with it a kind of trite cruelty; by looking for clues and demanding answers, I was inadvertently putting her on trial—all because I wanted some kind of verdict.[5] But her life was not some equation to be solved. She was a precious human being in a world that operates at random. We all are. And our subconscious need for control over ambiguity robs us of a kind of wholeness that should be valued above all else.

The empty ritual of the Effortless Perfection Myth pushes its followers onto a perceived path toward certainty that really just forces us to think in extremes—all or nothing, good or bad, safe or in peril. As we are consumed by it, we lose our tolerance for paradox, which is a problem because paradox is often at the core of the nuanced answers we are seeking to life's questions:[6]

- Failure leads to success.
- The only certainty is uncertainty.
- The only constant is change.

Locking ourselves into states of mind where these contradictions and complexities cannot exist in their fullness is a trap.

Releasing ourselves from this trap requires recognizing what the Indigo Girls put so wonderfully back in 1989: "the less I seek my source from some definitive, the closer I am to fine." In other (less lyrical) words, *the less we seek a false sense of certainty from misleading entities like the Effortless Perfection Myth, the closer we are to adapting healthier frames of mind that are able to comprehend the paradoxes of life.*

Furthermore, the less obsessively we chase after the perfect future, the more present in the now we become; and when we shift into recognizing the now as a legitimate and valuable place to be, we are able to more fully recognize the value of our already existing relationships, the accomplishments we have already reached, and the satisfaction we have already felt.

We become more open to making paradigm shifts in our modes of thinking and to redefining the meaning assigned to life experiences so the goal is no longer stockpiling future security, but taking a breath for long enough to consider the possibility that parts of life are already good. Bad things are bound to come our way, but if erroneously attempting to outwit the bad is no longer the central goal of our lives, we create space in our consciousness to feel the good of the now that our obsessive pursuits previously caused us to overlook and discount. We learn to take the good with the bad.

Since college, I've learned that I am just as much a paradox as the world is. As such, I am able to experience multiple truths at the same time. It is possible to feel overwhelmed and exuberant and anxious and unstoppable all at the same once because emotions are not things that need to be felt one at a time.

I've been the blissfully happy, peppy freshman who tented for over a month with friends to land a front-row seat at the UNC-Duke game where I screamed with electric excitement in unison with hundreds of my peers while fully painted blue. I've been the depressed sorority girl with an eating disorder crying herself to sleep because she didn't feel she belonged. I've been the focused student in the library realizing she might be developing a heart-fluttering crush on her study partner. I've been the abroad student awakened to the heartbreak of a life cut short, questioning the point of it all. I've been the inspired undergrad discovering her wildest passions and making career plans to follow them. And somehow all of these wildly different people are able to fit inside this one me.

Somehow, they fit inside each of us.

Chapter 42

Individually Overcoming the Myth by Rejecting Inflexible Thinking and Welcoming Uncertainty

I TOOK DISAPPOINTMENT HARD in college. The Effortless Perfection Myth had promised me that, if I followed its zeitgeist, I could expect results. So I did. I gave it my all and I developed an unhealthy, unrealistic expectation that college would no doubt be "the *best* four years of my life." Additionally, my concept of what I needed in order for it to be the best four years was not flexible. I'd yet to learn that expectations can turn into monsters if they are not kept in check.

Author Courtney Martin warns, "We are a generation of young women that were told they could *do anything* and heard they needed to *be everything*." I think I took that concept a step further, hearing: If you can *be everything*, you can expect to *lack nothing*. Thus, being and achieving everything on my list of lofty expectations became both my burden and my birthright.

I'd worked my butt off to get into the college I got into because I believed it was the place I'd be best set up to meet these expectations. I'd been praised as chock-full of potential; college was where I was cashing in all that potential. I mean, if I didn't reach my dream destiny, had all I'd gone through to make it to this point really been worth it? (This is where you, as a reader, should be registering impending disaster: *ALERT! ALERT! This girl's entitlement and inflexible thinking is not healthy. This ship is going down!)*

Down, down, down, indeed. Because possessing the *potential* for things to work out by no means ensures things *definitely will* work out. We are not owed success simply because we've set ourselves up (with a privileged amount of help and support, in my case) to reach it. To believe so would put one far over the line of what constitutes a healthy level of entitlement.

Furthermore, things "working out" can take on very different meanings. If you are *inflexible* in your picture of what a fulfilling college experience is meant to look like, you have a tiny window to make it through. But if you are open to *flexible* thought, to allowing your life to happen and trusting the meaning of different experiences to reveal themselves to you with time, that tiny window of fulfillment becomes a much larger door. *Flexible thinking asks just one thing in return—that we embrace or at least accept uncertainty,* for it knows what good can come from turning our fear of the unknown into a curiosity for it.

The Effortless Perfection Myth will, of course, fight us on this mindset change because it possesses a Machiavellian level of cunning. It prefers to encourage unadaptable, inflexible thinking because that, in turn, causes anxiety: "apprehension about future suffering—the fearful anticipation of an unbearable catastrophe one is hopeless to prevent."[1] That anxiety then threatens*: If you cannot make XYZ happen, then you will fail and suffer forever.* Opportunely, the Myth steps in: *See, you need me.* On and on, anxiety and the Myth feed each other via their ugly process of symbiosis.

Suddenly, we are seeing disaster and ruin at every turn, as the *possibility* of something going wrong becomes reason to believe that something *definitely will* go wrong. And that's when it's got you. That's when the Myth has you on your knees before it pleading: *Save me—you are my only hope.*

But surely, after having read all these pages in this book, you know it is most emphatically *not* the only hope. Surely, you've accumulated the knowledge you need to call Effortless Perfection out on its depression-inducing, highly gendered bullshit because you now understand that all that we are—our self-esteem, our confidence, our ability to be assertive and put ourselves out there, our capacity for both collective belonging and individual agency—is always evolving. To believe otherwise is to stagnate.

The Myth *wants* us to stagnate, to operate as though we can expect the world to be made of absolutes, of clear trades—you give it X and it gives you Y. But life is not always a fair trade, regardless of whatever agreement we think we've drawn up with the Effortless Perfection gods. Sometimes hard work and potential do not equal conventional success. Sometimes we give it everything and are still given a less-than-ideal hand of cards in return.

The Myth would have us looking at that hand, feeling paralyzed and cheated. Its inflexible thinking would have us in an anxious, arrogant, sorrowful state of self-pity: *How could this happen to me? I'm supposed to be on the VIP list!*

Pushing back against the Effortless Perfection Myth on an individual level is about throwing all that disingenuous crap out the window to make room for our own personal growth. It's about each of us adapting accordingly so that we don't, as author and self-help columnist Cheryl Strayed would put it, "surrender all [our] joy for an idea [we] used to have about [ourselves] that isn't true anymore."[2] We must let ourselves and our paths flexibly evolve.

Effortless Perfection makes you arrogant. Its false promises lift you high into the sky with your head among the clouds, when where you need to be to do your best work is down on the ground in the dirt with everyone else, struggling to blossom and become. If you want to push back against the Myth, you need to get your ass down here—down here is your salvation.

Looking back, my entire college career can be summed up in one word: recalculating. I plugged Effortless Perfection into my GPS and proceeded to run into an inordinate number of roadblocks and traffic delays. In the moment, I felt frustrated, but hindsight is 20/20 and, given time to reflect and be more flexible in my thinking about the meaning of various events, what was previously indignance has mostly turned into gratitude.

A running injury that kept me from participating in club sports forced me to find different extracurriculars, which led me to discover my passion for writing. An eating disorder led me to meet a psychologist who became a mentor for life and was instrumental in helping me down the road when I ran into an even greater struggle. The extra semester I needed to graduate gave me the opportunity to form closer bonds with three of the most inspiring and explorative friends I've ever known.

It took me a while to get over the initial disappointment—disappointment caused by the expectations I'd had for my college experience that never came to fruition. But what helped me move past that was recognizing just how much benefit I reaped from the detours I never intended to take and not letting that go unaccounted for. With time and perspective, I came to recognize that some of the richest gifts of my college experience were things I never even would have known to ask for.

Gretchen Rubin explains in *The Happiness Project*: "[T]he brain is stimulated by surprise, and successfully dealing with an unexpected situation gives a powerful sense of satisfaction. This is one of the many paradoxes of happiness: we seek to control our lives, but the unfamiliar and the unexpected are important sources of happiness."[3] Our most intense emotional responses are born out of moments that are "novel." We are happiest when we are growing. Becoming. Expanding our self-definition. Those things can only happen when we learn to welcome change and uncertainty and accept that we don't have all the answers.

Several of my interviewees experienced blessings in disguise during their college experiences, similar to my own. Aurora was particularly thankful for where her forced recalculations led her. As a second-semester senior, she was passed over for a job at McKinsey she had somewhat assumed she was destined for. Having been "hand-picked" her freshman year by older members of Vanderbilt student leadership and essentially "trained" to become student body president, this was the presumed next step since there was a "lineage of student body presidents and other Vandy alum working there [at McKinsey]." Even though she had made it to the final round, not getting an offer made her question herself deeply.

She was a known entity on campus. People expected great things from her. Graduating without a job lined up felt like a complete embarrassment. That is, until her perspective switched and it became "weirdly refreshing." Given the space to think outside a very narrowly defined pathway to success, Aurora was able to take a step back and think, "Okay, well, I wonder what it is I really like, since I guess I can try and do anything at this point." She now feels thankful that her original prayers went unanswered, since this opened an opportunity for her to follow a nontraditional path to the job she now has—a job she would not have even been able to dream up a description for two years prior.

Meanwhile, Charlotte hasn't quite managed to twist a happy ending onto her college experience, but she can at least look back and be proud of supporting herself through that hard time and making it to a better place. "Maybe it's okay this experience [of momentarily losing myself in college] happened when it happened and, if anything, it means I don't have to experience it later, and I can talk about it and give insight to others," she reflects. Going through the storm meant freeing herself from the demons of binge drinking and drugs and unhealthy relationships. Once on the other side, these things lost their power to control her. Acceptance of her struggles was humbling, whereas denial had been torturous.

Embracing uncertainty and replacing our fear of the unknown with a curiosity for it is obviously challenging. Those of us drawn to the pursuit of the Myth are not exactly wired to do so, but I believe we have the power to change and make updates to our motherboard. How? By asking ourselves the necessary questions and living out those questions, wherever and however far they take us.

Poet Rainer Maria Rilke writes, "Be patient toward all that is unsolved in your heart and try to love the questions themselves.... Do not now seek the answers, which cannot be given to you because you would not be able to live them. And the point is, to live everything. Live the questions now. Perhaps you will then gradually, without noticing it, live along some distant day into the answer."[4] His wise words urge us to leave room for uncertainty and mistakes, because there are some things we cannot just take someone else's word for—we need to have felt it and to know it in an incarnate way. It needs to be our own.

Sometimes that means walking into a mistake even if we know it is a mistake because personal experiences create nontransferable knowledge, and that knowledge is more valuable than being Effortlessly Perfect. Sometimes the wounds left by those mistakes evolve into gifts, if only we give them the space to do so.

The best pieces of who I've become are there in part because, as hard as I clung to the Myth for safety, it failed to protect me from all of which I was afraid. And thank God. Because my missteps made me more humble, my failures made my confidence more resilient, and my mistakes made me more empathetic. I am a better mentor and friend today because I've had the experiences necessary to connect with others when they most need me. We trust each other, in part, because we share some of the same wounds. We love each other, in part, because we are made of the same stuff.

If there is one life lesson I have taken away from college, it is this: *You can never label a moment as a good moment or a bad moment because that would imply finality.* As we continue adding more context to the narrative of our lives, specific moments often shift and morph their meanings all together. What may have felt like one of the worst things that happened to you while it was occurring could one day turn out to be the best. You just have to be willing to ride the wave all the way through—to watch relationships evolve, to experience desires changing and building, to push the emotional scope of what you thought it was possible to feel.

Chapter 43

Collectively Defeating the Myth by Embracing Vulnerability

THE EFFORTLESS PERFECTION MYTH THRIVES when people remain quiet about the various different ways they are impacted by it. It loves a tough exterior, a fake smile.

The Myth also makes it far too easy to accidentally play into its hands, because many of us want to be the friend whom others come to for help, while never asking for anything in return. We don't realize that this one-way flow of vulnerability is a total cop out. It impedes our ability to form closer relationships because what makes a bond truly special is the mutual trust that goes along with knowing you have both given each other a piece of yourselves. It takes courage to know that people can't hurt you if you don't give them your heart, but to give them that power anyway.

Having another share a vulnerability with us can be one of the most incredibly freeing and gratifying experiences. To me, it means I have comported myself in a way that has earned their trust. After all, the word "vulnerability" comes from the Latin word "to wound," thus to be vulnerable is to make oneself open to being wounded. To have another share a secret with you that gives you that kind of power, and trust you will not use it against them—I think that is the greatest possible sign of love and respect we can ever hope to receive. It shows we have achieved something infinitely better than Effortless Perfection. We have achieved being the kind of person who grants others the feeling that, when they are in our presence, they are safe to be their fullest, most honest selves. What an incredible gift to be able to offer, and what an incredible gift to receive.

Of course, there are limits to the manner in which we should be participating in this kind of sharing. Vulnerability requires mutual respect and boundaries. Feelings and experiences that are still raw or maintain a fragility about them should only be shared with those who have earned the privilege of hearing them. Purging is not vulnerability. Oversharing is not vulnerability. Blindly throwing our fears and struggles out into the open hoping someone will catch them is not only risky, but it can be selfish. We can't thrust our fears onto strangers in the hope we will no longer need to lug them around ourselves.

Instead, we should be treating our vulnerabilities tenderly and preciously. They are the strongest tools we possess for creating bonds. Studies show that connecting with others while experiencing stress causes the release of oxytocin, the so-called "bonding hormone,"[1] which is our body's way of showing us it wants us to respond to stress by connecting in loving and comforting relationships.

The best kind of vulnerability occurs as a give-and-take. We take turns holding each other up in our moments of weakness, so that neither person ever has to feel alone. Sharing our struggles allows us to take them on as a team. And when we recognize the interconnectedness of the struggles we face, we can even rally behind those social issues and political concerns as a force for change.

I felt compelled to write this book because of the countless times I found myself pushing past the Effortless Perfection Myth, past the dominant narrative, past the presentation of false self to reveal that I was struggling with something, only to have my confidants reply that they were struggling with that same thing too, especially my female peers. The toxic trends we faced—whether in relation to self-esteem, confidence, assertiveness, body image, hookup culture, and belonging—were undeniable. Everyone was trying their best to slyly navigate their way through them, but nobody I knew had escaped unscathed.

Putting this book together was about doing more than recognizing the similarities in our situations. It was about working together to break down the structural issues of our society, specifically on college campuses, that were bringing about such painful side effects. I am forever grateful to the numerous interviewees who were willing to share some of their deepest vulnerabilities with me so that I could do exactly that.

Every time I hung up the phone after a two-hour-plus call or closed my notebook after a lengthy in-person meeting, a sense of affirmation would wash over me. We were doing it! We were denying the Effortless Perfection Myth its power! Every story shared was a different young woman saying, "My shame will not own me. My fears of rejection will not control me. I can overcome."

Owning our stories and the baggage that comes along with them can be hard, but when we use them to mobilize into a force of collective action, the accompanying sense of purpose is the most empowering force I know. All it takes is giving up the impossible pursuit of Effortless Perfection, so that we can then take up the mantle of being a person who allows others to feel seen, heard, and valued.

A great way to start this conversation is going to my website (www.caralenapeterson.com) and downloading the resource entitled "Questions for Starting an Internal and/or Group Dialogue about Effortless Perfection." This bonus material provides a pointed, in-depth series of prompts breaking down each chapter of this book so conversations can more easily occur in our classrooms, dorm rooms, and family dinner tables.

The most important step colleges and universities can take to combat the Effortless Perfection Myth, other than providing ample mental health resources on their campuses, is to support student efforts to tell their stories. The dominant narrative of Effortless Perfection (discussed near the start of this book in Chapter 3) needs to be challenged with more honest, alternative narratives that recognize struggle as normal and healthy (discussed in Chapter 4).

Luckily, a small but growing body of campaigns and organizations has already begun to take up this torch.

> *#HalftheStory* encourages individuals to "share parts of their lives that exist outside of the standard social media" by posting more than just a highlight reel of their best moments and, instead, bringing up taboo issues like mental health and belonging as well.
>
> The *What I Be Project* creates photo campaigns, often on college campuses, that allow individuals to highlight their insecurities while also using their own words to frame those stories the way they want them to be told.
>
> *Me Too Monologues*, established at Duke roughly a decade before the #MeToo movement, curates a theatrical performance of monologues that students write and submit anonymously about struggles with identity issues like race, gender, sexuality, socioeconomic status, mental health, religion, and ability. The program has spread to multiple other university campuses due to its national expansion campaign.
>
> The *Madison Holleran Foundation* strives to prepare high school seniors and college freshmen for what is often a difficult transition period in their lives by bringing in speakers to shed light on mental health challenges that may befall

> them. The foundation also strives "to prevent suicides and assist those in a crisis situation with resources that will aid them during their time of need" and to support "survivors of suicide, the loved ones struggling to deal and cope with these heartbreaking tragedies and the unanswered questions that are commonly left behind."

Each of these platforms and organizations, along with many others like them, is eager for more engagement. They strive to encourage undergrads to show enough of their own vulnerabilities that others do not feel the need to hide their own. If we want to push back against the Effortless Perfection Myth and the mental health crisis it has helped to create on college campuses, institutions all across the U.S. need to create and support vital efforts such as these.

I challenge us all to find ways to implement such changes on our campuses and in our communities.

References

Introduction

1. Lopez, Mark Hugo, and Ana Gonzalez-Barrera. "Women's College Enrollment Gains Leave Men Behind." *Pew Research Center*, March 6, 2014. https://www.pewresearch.org/fact-tank/2014/03/06/womens-college-enrollment-gains-leave-men-behind.

Chapter 1

1. Roth, Susan, Nannerl Keohane, Donna Lisker, Ann Brown, Robin A. Burke, Sally M. Dickinson, Allison Haltom, et al. Women's Initiative: Duke University. Duke Publications Group, 2003. http://universitywomen.law.stanford.edu/reports/WomensInitiativeReport.pdf.
2. Anonymous. "Effortless Perfection?" *Chronicle*, Duke University. October 23, 2003. Accessed May 2015.

Chapter 3

1. Simmons, Rachel. *Enough as She Is: How to Help Girls Move beyond Impossible Standards of Success to Live Healthy, Happy, and Fulfilling Lives*, 157. New York: Harper, 2019.
2. Melanie, Joy. "Speaking Truth to Power: Understanding the Dominant, Animal-Eating Narrative for Vegan Empowerment and Social Transformation." *One Green Planet*, January 21, 2013.

3. "What Is Groupthink." studylib.net. https://studylib.net/doc/8345019/what-is-groupthink. Accessed July 31, 2021.

4. Ibid.

Chapter 4

1. Bamberg, Michael. "C*onsidering Counter Narratives." Considering Counter-Narratives Studies in Narrative Narrating, Resisting, Making Sense*, 2004, 351–71. https://doi.org/10.1075/sin.4.43bam.

2. Ibid.

3. Zernike, Kate. "Ease Up, Top Colleges Tell Stressed Applicants." *New York Times*, December 7, 2000. https://www.nytimes.com/2000/12/07/us/ease-up-top-colleges-tell-stressed-applicants.html.

4. Brown, Brené. *Daring Greatly: How the Courage to Be Vulnerable Transforms the Way We Live, Love, Parent, and Lead*, 28. London: Penguin Books, 2015.

5. @arianaspringflower. "To Many People, I'm the over Achiever." @HalfTheStory. Instagram, November 8, 2015. https://www.instagram.com/p/91cnPHEXE9/.

6. @lucmaloney. "I've Always Been Known as the Athletic Girl." @HalfTheStory. Instagram, November 16, 2015. https://www.instagram.com/p/-JmBsOEXB1/

7. @jacqbouchil. "I Go to the University of Southern California and Spent My First Semester Abroad in Paris." @HalfTheStory. Instagram, August 1, 2016. https://www.instagram.com/p/BIkPygQB6ts/.

8. @lanesha_reagan. "In High School I Always Felt like I Had to Put a Mask on." @HalfTheStory. Instagram, August 21, 2017. https://www.instagram.com/p/BYE4nmGn4n4/.

9. Quindlen, Anna. Essay. Being Perfect, 15. New York: Random House, 2005.

Chapter 5

1. Steinem, Gloria. *Revolution from Within: A Book of Self-Esteem*, 3. Boston: Little, Brown and Co., 1992.
2. Ibid, 6.
3. Ibid, 8.
4. Fissinger, Mary Rose. "Female BC Students Report Lower Self-Confidence When Leaving College." *Heights*, Boston College Newspapers, February 25, 2013. https://newspapers.bc.edu/?a=d&d=bcheights20130225-01.2.6&e=-------en-20--1--txt-txIN-------.
5. "Self-Esteem." Merriam-Webster. https://www.merriam-webster.com/dictionary/self-esteem. Accessed August 28, 2021.
6. Kay, Katty, and Claire Shipman. *The Confidence Code: The Science and Art of Self-Assurance—What Women Should Know*, 51. New York: HarperBusiness, 2018.

Chapter 6

1. Russell, Michelle. "What Holds Us Back: Is Confidence as Important as Competence in the Workplace?" PCMA Convene, June 1, 2014. http://www.pcmaconvene.org/features/what-holds-us-back-is-confidence-as-important-as-competence-in-the-workplace/.
2. Babcock, Linda, and Sara Laschever. *Women Don't Ask: Negotiation and the Gender Divide*. Princeton, NJ: Princeton University Press, 2003.
3. Chaudhry, Lakshmi. "The Supergirl Syndrome." *Nation*, May 1, 2007.https://www.thenation.com/article/archive/supergirl-syndrome.
4. Ibid.
5. Ibid.
6. Ibid.
7. Spar, Debora L. *Wonder Women: Sex, Power, and the Quest for Perfection*, 169–70. New York: Farrar, Straus, and Giroux, 2013.

8. Ibid.
9. Ibid.
10. Ibid.
11. Quindlen, *Being Perfect*, 15.

Chapter 7

1. Geary, David. "Women's Advantages in Social Cognition: An Evolved Change?" *Psychology Today*, October 23, 2019. https://www.psychologytoday.com/us/blog/male-female/201910/women-s-advantages-in-social-cognition.
2. Nolen-Hoeksema, Susan. *Women Who Think Too Much: How to Break Free of Overthinking and Reclaim Your Life*, 103. London: Piatkus, 2004.
3. Ibid, 104.
4. Ferguson, Tamara J., and Susan L. Crowley. "Gender Differences in the Organization of Guilt and Shame." *Sex Roles*. 37 (July 1997): 19–44. https://link.springer.com/article/10.1023/A:1025684502616.
5. Brown, Brené. *The Gifts of Imperfection: Let Go of Who You Think You Are Supposed to Be and Embrace Who You Are*, 39. Minneapolis: Hazelden, 2010.
6. Ibid, 68.
7. Ibid.
8. Quindlen, *Being Perfect*, 32.
9. Brown, *Gifts of Imperfection*, 11.

Chapter 9

1. Kay and Shipman, *Confidence Code*, 42.
2. Ibid, 50.

3. Kay, Katty, and Claire Shipman. "Preface to the 2018 Edition." *The Confidence Code: The Science and Art of Self-Assurance—What Women Should Know*, xi. New York: HarperBusiness, 2018.

4. "The Greek Culture Initiative: Report on Gender and Greek Experience." *Chronicle*, Duke University, 2013. http://archive.dukechronicle.com/gci-report.pdf.

5. Gentile, Brittany, Shelly Grabe, Brenda Dolan-Pascoe, Jean M. Twenge, Brooke E. Wells, and Alissa Maitino. "Gender Differences in Domain-Specific Self-Esteem: A Meta-Analysis." *Review of General Psychology* 13, no. 1 (2009): 34–45. https://doi.org/10.1037/a0013689.

6. "The Greek Culture Initiative."

7. Roberts, Emily. "Is College to Blame for Low Self-Esteem in Women?" *Healthy Place: America's Mental Health Channel*, October 2013. https://www.healthyplace.com/blogs/buildingselfesteem/2013/10/is-college-to-blame-for-low-self-esteem-in-women.

8. Simmons, *Enough as She Is*, 141.

9. Deresiewicz, William. "Don't Send Your Kid to the Ivy League." *Nation*, July 22, 2014. https://newrepublic.com/article/118747/ivy-league-schools-are-overrated-send-your-kids-elsewhere.

10. Ibid.

Chapter 10

1. Deresiewicz, "Don't Send Your Kid to the Ivy League."

2. Kay and Shipman, *The Confidence Code*, 123.

Chapter 11

1. Hinshaw, Stephen P., and Rachel Kranz. *The Triple Bind: Saving Our Teenage Girls from Today's Pressures*, 64. New York: Ballantine Books, 2009.

2. Ibid.

3. Ibid.

4. Rampell, Catherine. "The Great Grade Deflation Experiment, STEM vs. Humanities." The Washington Post. WP Company, October 26, 2021. https://www.washingtonpost.com/news/rampage/wp/2014/08/12/the-great-grade-deflation-experiment-stem-vs-humanities/.

5. Rampell, Catherine. "Women Shouldn't Chase after A's in College to Make More Later." *Washington Post*, March 10, 2014. https://www.washingtonpost.com/opinions/catherine-rampell-women-should-embrace-the-bs-in-college-to-make-more-later/2014/03/10/1e15113a-a871-11e3-8d62-419db477a0e6_story.html.

6. Ibid.

7. Orrell, Brent, and Daniel Cox. "Blacks, Latinos Feel Unwelcome in STEM Careers. And That's a Big Problem for Our Economy." *USA Today*. July 28, 2020. https://www.usatoday.com/story/opinion/2020/07/28/why-women-minorities-still-feel-excluded-stem-careers-column/5516913002/.

8. Rampell. "Women Shouldn't Chase after A's."

9. Fuller, Jessica. "The Duke 'Blah' Factor." *Chronicle*. Duke University, December 4, 2007. https://www.dukechronicle.com/article/2007/12/duke-blah-factor.

10. Kay and Shipman, *Confidence Code*, 106.

11. Ibid.

Chapter 12

1. "Stereotype Threat." National Institutes of Health. U.S. Department of Health and Human Services. https://diversity.nih.gov/sociocultural-factors/stereotype-threat. Accessed August 28, 2021.

2. Ibid.

3. Ibid.

4. Severiens, Sabine, and Geert ten Dam. "Leaving College: A Gender Comparison in Male and Female-Dominated Programs." *Research in Higher Education* 53 (2012): 453–70. https://link.springer.com/article/10.1007/s11162-011-9237-0.

5. "Researchers Find Confidence Is Key to Women's Spatial Skills." News and Events. University of Warwick. December 5, 2011. https://warwick.ac.uk/newsandevents/pressreleases/researchers_find_confidence/.

6. Azar, Beth. "Math + Culture = Gender Gap?" *American Psychological Association* 41, no. 7 (2010): 40.

7. Sandberg, Sheryl, and Nell Scovell. *Lean In: Women, Work, and the Will to Lead*, 28. New York: Knopf, 2013.

8. Mohr, Tara Sophia. "Why Women Don't Apply for Jobs Unless They're 100% Qualified." *Harvard Business Review*, March 8, 2021. https://hbr.org/2014/08/why-women-dont-apply-for-jobs-unless-theyre-100-qualified.

9. Bahn, Kate. Faking It: Women, Academia, and Impostor Syndrome." *Vitae*, May 2, 2015. https://chroniclevitae.com/news/412-faking-it-women-academia-and-imposter-syndrome.

10. Rosette, Ashleigh Shelby, and Robert W. Livingston. "Failure Is Not an Option for Black Women: Effects of Organizational Performance on Leaders with Single versus Dual-Subordinate Identities." *Journal of Experimental Social Psychology* 48, no. 5 (September 2012): 1162–67. https://doi.org/10.1016/j.jesp.2012.05.002.

11. Ibid.

12. Ibid.

13. Furnham, A. "Self-Estimates of Intelligence: Culture and Gender Difference in Self and Other Estimates of Both General (G) and Multiple Intelligences." *Personality and Individual Differences* 31, no. 8 (December 2001): 1381–1405. https://doi.org/10.1016/s0191-8869(00)00232-4.

14. Damour, Lisa. "Why Girls Beat Boys at School and Lose to Them at the Office." *New York Times*. February 7, 2019. https://www.nytimes.com/2019/02/07/opinion/sunday/girls-school-confidence.html.

Chapter 13

1. Chamorro-Premuzic, Tomas. "Why Do so Many Incompetent Men Become Leaders?" *Harvard Business Review*, November 26, 2019. https://hbr.org/2013/08/why-do-so-many-incompetent-men.
2. Miller, Claire Cain. "The Problem for Women Is Not Winning. It's Deciding to Run." *New York Times*, October 25, 2016. https://www.nytimes.com/2016/10/25/upshot/the-problem-for-women-is-not-winning-its-deciding-to-run.html.
3. Ibid.
4. Johnson, Jenna. "On College Campuses, a Gender Gap in Student Government." *Washington Post*, March 16, 2011. https://www.washingtonpost.com/local/education/on-college-campuses-a-gender-gap-in-student-government/2011/03/10/ABim1Bf_story.html.
5. Lawless, Jennifer L., and Richard L. Fox. Rep. *Girls Just Wanna Not Run*. Women & Politics Institute, March 2013. https://www.american.edu/spa/wpi/upload/girls-just-wanna-not-run_policy-report.pdf.
6. New, Jake. "Getting Women to Run." *Inside Higher Ed*, November 4, 2014. https://www.insidehighered.com/news/2014/11/04/female-students-still-scarce-student-government-executive-positions.
7. "History of Women Governors." CAWP, March 3, 2021. http://www.cawp.rutgers.edu/history-women-governors.
8. Blazina, Carrie, and Drew DeSilver. "A Record Number of Women Are Serving in the 117th Congress." Pew Research Center. Pew Research Center, January 22, 2021. https://www.pewresearch.org/fact-tank/2021/01/15/a-record-number-of-women-are-serving-in-the-117th-congress/.
9. "History of Women of Color in U.S. Politics." CAWP, July 8, 2021. http://www.cawp.rutgers.edu/history-women-color-us-politics.
10. Ibid.
11. Newsom, Jennifer Siebel. *Miss Representation*. United States: Girls' Club Entertainment, 2011.

12. Malone, Clare, and Julia Azari. "Thinking They're 'Unqualified' Is a Big Reason More Women Don't Run for Office." *FiveThirtyEight*. ESPN, April 8, 2016. https://fivethirtyeight.com/features/why-calling-hillary-clinton-unqualified-smacks-of-sexism/.

13. Chemaly, Soraya. "The Credibility Gap: How Sexism Shapes Human Knowledge | Soraya Chemaly | TEDxBarcelonaWwomen." *TEDx*. YouTube, July 28, 2015. https://www.youtube.com/watch?v=HJqtUUDhaxA.

14. Ibid.

Chapter 14

1. Chemaly, Soraya. *Rage Becomes Her: The Power of Women's Anger*, 16. New York: Atria Books, 2019.

2. Kay and Shipman, *Confidence Code*, 194.

3. Bowles, Hannah Riley, Linda Babcock, and Kathleen L. McGinn. "Constraints and Triggers: Situational Mechanics of Gender in Negotiation." *Journal of Personality and Social Psychology* 89, no. 6 (2005): 951–65. https://doi.org/10.1037/0022-3514.89.6.951.

Chapter 15

1. McGinn, Kathleen L., and Nicole Tempest. "Heidi Roizen." Harvard Business School Case 800-228, January 2000. (Revised April 2010.) https://www.hbs.edu/faculty/Pages/item.aspx?num=26880.

2. Ibid.

3. Babcock and Laschever. *Women Don't Ask*, 22.

4. Ibid.

5. Ibid, 20.

6. Claridge, Tristan. "Social Sanctions: Overview, Meaning, Examples, Types and Importance." Social Capital Research, February 12, 2020. https://www.socialcapitalresearch.com/social-sanctions/.

7. Babcock and Laschever. *Women Don't Ask*, 12.

8. Jakobson, Haley. "December 22nd, 2016." *Write Like Prayers*. Self-published, 2018.

Chapter 16

1. Steinem, *Revolution from Within*, 114.
2. Thompson, Martine. "How I Learned to Stop Being a 'Chill Girl' and Start Being Me." *Vogue*, September 12, 2017. https://www.vogue.com/article/how-to-let-go-of-chill-girl-persona.
3. Ibid.
4. Ibid.
5. Cordero, Daniella. "I Need Feminism Because I Don't Want to Have to Apologize For My Strong Opinions." Photo posted to Facebook. Durham, NC: *Who Needs Feminism Campaign*, April 10, 2012. https://www.facebook.com/WhoNeeds Feminism / photos/a.148163118645642/148163955312225. Accessed August 28, 2021.
6. "Who Needs Feminism?" Tumblr. http://whoneedsfeminism.tumblr.com/. Accessed 2016.

Chapter 17

1. Chemaly, *Rage Becomes Her*, xvii.
2. Engel, Beverly. *The Nice Girl Syndrome: Stop Being Manipulated and Abused and Start Standing up for Yourself*, 169. Hoboken, NJ: Wiley, 2010.
3. Ibid, 167.
4. Ibid, 177.
5. Brown, *Gifts of Imperfection*, 16.
6. Ibid, 17.
7. Ibid.

Chapter 18

1. Fey, Tina. *Bossypants*, 77. New York: Little, Brown and Company, 2013.
2. Crosley, Sloane. "Why Women Apologize and Should Stop." *New York Times*. June 22, 2015. https://www.nytimes.com/2015/06/23/opinion/when-an-apology-is-anything-but.html.
3. Vrabel, Ani. "The Simple Phrase I Had to Banish from My Vocabulary." *Huffington Post*, May 31, 2014. http://www.huffingtonpost.com/ani-vrabel/stop-apologizing-im-not-sorry_b_5021125.html.
4. Xiao, Yao. "If You Want to Say 'Thank You,' Don't Say 'Sorry.'" *BoredPanda.com*, January 2016. https://www.boredpanda.com/stop-saying-sorry-say-thank-you-comic-yao-xiao/?utm_source=google&utm_medium=organic&utm_campaign=organic.
5. Udwadia, Zarah, and Roma Sonik. "Lizete Dos Santos, #noapologies for my authority." Photo posted to Facebook. Durham, NC: Duke Baldwin Scholars No Apologies Campaign, November 14, 2014. https://m.facebook.com/noapologiesdukeuniversity/photos/a.1467609690181845/1467752230167591/?type=3&source=54&ref=page_internal. Accessed April 7, 2016).
6. Udwadia, Zarah, and Roma Sonik. "Adesuwa Giwa-Osagie, #noapologies for My Space." Photo posted to Facebook. Durham, NC: Duke Baldwin Scholars No Apologies Campaign, November 14, 2014. https://m.facebook.com/noapologiesdukeuniversity/photos/a.1467609690181845/1469686449974169/?type=3&source=54&ref=page_internal. Accessed April 7, 2016).
7. Udwadia, Zarah, and Roma Sonik. "Dr. Heekyoung Hahn, #noapologies for my Ambitions." Photo posted to Facebook. Durham, NC: Duke Baldwin Scholars No Apologies Campaign, November 14, 2014. https://m.facebook.com/noapologiesdukeuniversity/photos/a.1467609690181845/1467736030169211/?type=3&source=54&ref=page_internal. Accessed April 7, 2016).
8. "Pantene 'Sorry, Not Sorry' Commercial." YouTube. Cause Marketing, March 11, 2017. https://www.youtube.com/watch?v=TcGKxLJ4ZGI.

9. Cauterucci, "New Chrome App Helps Women Stop Saying 'Just' and 'Sorry' in Emails." *Slate Magazine*. Slate, December 29, 2015. https://slate.com/human-interest/2015/12/new-chrome-app-helps-women-stop-saying-just-and-sorry-in-emails.html.

Chapter 19

1. Babcock and Laschever, *Women Don't Ask*, 70.
2. Ibid.
3. Ibid.
4. Ibid.
5. Major, B., McFarlin, D. B., & Gagnon, D. (1984). Overworked and underpaid: On the nature of gender differences in personal entitlement. *Journal of Personality and Social Psychology*, 47(6), 1399–1412.
6. Jost, John T. "An Experimental Replication of the Depressed-Entitlement Effect among Women." *Psychology of Women Quarterly*21, no. 3 (1997): 387–93. https://doi.org/10.1111/j.1471-6402.1997.tb00120.x.
7. Najumi, Mohadesa. "Why the Woman Who Does Not Require Validation from Anyone Is the Most Feared Individual on the Planet." *HuffPost UK*, May 15, 2014. https://www.huffingtonpost.co.uk/mohadesa-najumi/ban-bossy-women-who-do-not-need-validation-are-feared_b_4971919.html.
8. Steinem, *Revolution from Within*, 53.

Chapter 20

1. Kurth, Candace L., Dean D. Krahn, Karen Nairn, and Adam Drewnowski. "The Severity of Dieting and Bingeing Behaviors in College Women: Interview Validation of Survey Data." *Journal of Psychiatric Research* 29, no. 3 (1995): 211–25. https://doi.org/10.1016/0022-3956(95)00002-m.

2. Mintz, Laurie B., and Nancy E. Betz. “Prevalence and Correlates of Eating Disordered Behaviors among Undergraduate Women.” *Journal of Counseling Psychology*35, no. 4 (1988): 463–71. https://doi.org/10.1037/0022-0167.35.4.463.

3. Shisslak, Catherine M., Marjorie Crago, and Linda S. Estes. “The Spectrum of Eating Disturbances.” *International Journal of Eating Disorders*18 (1995): 209219. https://doi.org/10.1002/1098-108X(199511)18:3<209::AID-EAT22601803 03>3.0.CO;2-E.

4. Shisslak, Crao, and Estes, “The Spectrum of Eating Disturbances.”

5. Castle, Kathryn S., “Attachment, Wellness, and Disordered Eating in College Women.” *Counseling and Human Services—Dissertations*4 (2008). https://surface.syr.edu/chs_etd/4.

6. Berko, Katherine, “*The Pressure to Be Thin: Examining Eating Disorders and the Duke Culture that Contributes to Them.*” *Chronicle*, Duke University. November 29, 2017.

7. Noordenbos, Greta, Anna Oldenhave, Jennifer Muschter, and Nynke Terpstra. “Characteristics and Treatment of Patients with Chronic Eating Disorders.” *Eating Disorders*10, no. 1 (2002): 15–29. https://doi.org/10.1080/106402602753573531.

8. Martin, Courtney E. *Perfect Girls, Starving Daughters: How the Quest for Perfection Is Harming Young Women*, 26. New York: Berkley Books, 2008.

9. Castle, “Attachment, Wellness, and Disordered Eating in College.”

10. Grigg, Margaret, Jenny Bowman, and Sally Redman. “Disordered Eating and Unhealthy Weight Reduction Practices among Adolescent Females.” *Preventive Medicine*25, no. 6 (1996): 748–56. https://doi.org/10.1006/pmed.1996.0115.

11. Castle, “Attachment, Wellness, and Disordered Eating in College Women.”

12. Simmons, *Enough as She Is*, 63.

13. "Body Dysmorphic Disorder." Mayo Clinic. Mayo Foundation for Medical Education and Research, October 29, 2019. http://www.mayoclinic.org/diseases-conditions/body-dysmorphic-disorder/basics/definition/con-20029953.

Chapter 21

1. West, Lindy. *Shrill: Notes from a Loud Woman,* 76. New York: Hachette, 2016.

Chapter 22

1. "Gender Inequality in Film—An Infographic." *New York Film Academy Blog.* New York Film Academy, November 25, 2013.
2. Goode, Erica. "Study Finds Tv Alters Fiji Girls' View of Body." *New York Times,* May 20, 1999. https://www.nytimes.com/1999/05/20/world/study-finds-tv-alters-fiji-girls-view-of-body.html.
3. Ibid.
4. Ibid.
5. Jhally, Sut. *Dream Worlds 3: Desire, Sex & Power in Music Video.* 2007; Media Education Foundation. Transcript.
6. Daw, Stephen. "10 Popular Music Videos That Feature Porn Stars." *Billboard,* 14 Mar. 2018, https://www.billboard.com/articles/news/pride/8247018/music-videos-porn-stars-taylor-swift/.
7. Valenti, Jessica. *He's a Stud, She's a Slut, and 49 Other Double Standards Every Woman Should Know,* 166. New York: Seal Press, 2008.
8. Guttmann, A. "U.S. Advertising Spending 2015–2022." *Statista,* March 28, 2019. https://www.statista.com/statistics/272314/advertising-spending-in-the-us/.
9. Lovett, Edward. "Most Models Meet Criteria for Anorexia, Size 6 Is Plus Size: Magazine." *ABC News.* ABC News Network, January 13, 2012. http://abcnews.go.com/blogs/headlines/2012/01/most-models-meet-criteria-for-anorexia-size-6-is-plus-size-magazine/.

10. Wolf, Naomi. *The Beauty Myth: How Images of Female Beauty Are Used against Women*, 65. New York: W. Morrow, 1991.

11. Goldman, Robert, Deborah Heath, and Sharon L. Smith. "Commodity Feminism." *Critical Studies in Mass Communication* 8, no. 3 (1991): 333–51. https://doi.org/10.1080/15295039109366801.

12. Wolf, *The Beauty Myth*,65.

13. Ibid, 66.

14. Ibid.

15. Ibid, 10.

16. Gaesser, G. *Big Fat Lies: The Truth About Your Weight and Your Health*. New York: Fawcett Columbine, 1996.

17. Newsom, *Miss Representation*

Chapter 23

1. Koul, Scacchi. *One Day We'll All Be Dead and None of This Will Matter: Essays*, 179. London: Picador, 2017.

2. Knapp, Caroline. *Appetites:* Why Women Want. Berkeley, CA: Counterpoint, 2012.

3. Tsai, Ashley and Sarah McCaffery. Photos posted on Facebook. Durham, NC: Duke WHO Speaks campaign, November 27, 2012. https://www.facebook.com/whospeaks/. Accessed March 20, 2016: "DO YOU EAT?" "TOO BIG/TOO SMALL." "MAN MUSCLES." "SKINNY B*TCH." "YOUR THIGHS SHOULD NOT BE TOUCHING."

4. Wolf, *Beauty Myth*, 281–82.

5. Simmons, *Enough as She Is*, 65.

6. Jacobson, Rae. "College Students and Eating Disorders." Child Mind Institute, May 18, 2021. https://childmind.org/article/eating-disorders-and-college/.

Chapter 24

1. Simmons, *Enough as She Is*, 64.

2. Ibid, 64–65.

3. Frey, William H. "The US Will Become 'Minority White' in 2045, Census Projects." Brookings, September 10, 2018. https://www.brookings.edu/blog/the-avenue/2018/03/14/the-us-will-become-minority-white-in-2045-census-projects/.

4. D., Elle. "Why Google's Images of Professional vs Unprofessional Styles Aren't as Racist as You Think." BGLH Marketplace, December 28, 2017. http://blackgirllonghair.com/2016/04/why-googles-images-of-professional-vs-unprofessional-styles-arent-as-racist-as-you-think/.

Chapter 25

1. "Roth, Geneen. "WOMEN, WEIGHT AND POWER: Releasing the Energy of Obsession." Geneen Roth, October 12, 2018. https://geneenroth.com/workshops/three-keys-to-vitality-radiance-and-weight-loss/#.

Chapter 26

1. "Eating Disorder Statistics." *Gen Psych*, October 17, 2020. https://www.genpsych.com/post/eating-disorder-statistics.

2. Knapp, Caroline. *Appetites*, 90.

3. "Eating Disorder Statistics." *Gen Psych*.

4. Castle. "Attachment, Wellness, and Disordered Eating in College Women."

5. Knapp, *Appetites*, 129.

6. Keller, Kathleen, Samantha Kling, Bari Fuchs, Alaina Pearce, Nicole Reigh, Travis Masterson, and Kara Hickok. "A Biopsychosocial Model of Sex Differences in Children's Eating Behaviors." *Nutrients* 11, no. 3 (2019): 682. https://doi.org/10.3390/nu11030682.

7. Simmons, *Enough as She Is*, 60.

8. Martin, *Perfect Girls, Starving Daughters*, 23.

9. Ibid.

Chapter 27

1. Knapp, *Appetites*, 167.

2. Arcelus, Jon, Alex J. Mitchell, Jackie Wales, and Søren Nielsen. "Mortality Rates in Patients with Anorexia Nervosa and Other Eating Disorders." *Archives of General Psychiatry* 68, no. 7 (2011): 724. https://doi.org/10.1001/archgenpsychiatry.2011.74.

3. Sullivan, P. F. "Mortality in Anorexia Nervosa." *American Journal of Psychiatry* 152, no. 7 (1995): 1073–74. https://doi.org/10.1176/ajp.152.7.1073.

4. Young, Iris Marion. Essay. *On Female Body Experience: "Throwing like a Girl" and Other Essays*, 32. Oxford: Oxford University Press, 2005.

5. "Picture of Sign below Scale at Denver Center for Bariatric Surgery—Michael A. Sayder Quote: This Scale Can Only Give You a Numerical Reflection of Your Relationship with Gravity. That's It." loveforquotes.com. https://loveforquotes.com/i/8d4f7d55f4114e9abf79a8f2240bfccb. Accessed August 28, 2021.

Chapter 28

1. Freitas, Donna. *The End of Sex: How Hookup Culture Is Leaving a Generation Unhappy, Sexually Unfulfilled, and Confused about Intimacy*, 21. New York: Basic Books, 2013.

2. Ibid, 176.

Chapter 29

1. Williams, Alex. "The End of Courtship?" *New York Times*, January 11, 2013. https://www.nytimes.com/2013/01/13/fashion/the-end-of-courtship.html.

2. Narin, Jordana. "No Labels, No Drama, Right?" *New York Times*, April 30, 2015. https://www.nytimes.com/2015/05/03/style/modern-love-college-essay-winner.html.

3. Duke Student Broadcasting. "Hook-up Culture—Shaina Lubliner | Me Too Monologues." YouTube. March 21, 2018. Recorded theater performance, 9:10. https://www.youtube.com/watch?v=72J82_3upgE&index=4&list=PLNxqB7I9iGR-CzcLRJaV2VzC_sKUaUAEm.

4. Ibid.

5. Ibid.

6. Spar, *Wonder Women*, 74.

7. LaBrie, Joseph W., Justin F. Hummer, Tehniat M. Ghaidarov, Andrew Lac, and Shannon R. Kenney. "Hooking up in the College Context: The Event-Level Effects of Alcohol Use and Partner Familiarity on Hookup Behaviors and Contentment." *Journal of Sex Research* 51, no. 1 (2012): 62–73. https://doi.org/10.1080/00224499.2012.714010.

8. Glass, Gary. 'Sexual Entitlement on Campus." Email, 2015.

9. Ibid.

10. Ibid.

Chapter 30

1. Reitman, Janet. "Sex & Scandal at Duke." *Rolling Stone*, June 25, 2018. https://www.rollingstone.com/culture/culture-news/sex-scandal-at-duke-113674/.

2. Lawson, Richard. "Duke Frats Send Charming Halloween Party Invitations to Coeds." *Gawker*. https://www.gawker.com/5680541/duke-frats-send-charming-halloween-party-invitations-to-coeds. Accessed August 2, 2021.

3. Ibid.

4. Levy, Ariel. *Female Chauvinist Pigs: Women and the Rise of Raunch Culture*, 39. London: Simon & Schuster, 2006.

5. Ibid.
6. Reitman, "Sex & Scandal at Duke."
7. Ibid.
8. Ibid.
9. Ibid.
10. Ibid.
11. Ibid.
12. Ibid.

Chapter 31

1. Reitman, "Sex & Scandal at Duke."
2. Ibid.
3. Birger, Jon. *Date-Onomics: How Dating Became a Lopsided Numbers Game*. New York: Workman, 2016.
4. Uecker, Jeremy E, and Mark D Regnerus. "Bare Market: Campus Sex Ratios, Romantic Relationships, and Sexual Behavior." *Sociological Quarterly* 51, no. 3 (2010): 408–35. https://www.ncbi.nlm.nih.gov/pmc/articles/PMC3130599/.
5. Ibid.

Chapter 32

1. McClelland, Sara I. "Intimate Justice: A Critical Analysis of Sexual Satisfaction." *Social and Personality Psychology Compass*4, no. 9 (2010): 663–80. https://doi.org/10.1111/j.1751-9004.2010.00293.x.
2. Orenstein, Peggy. "What Young Women Believe about Their Own Sexual Pleasure." TED, October 2016. https://www.ted.com/talks/peggy_orenstein_what_young_women_believe_about_their_own_sexual_pleasure/transcript?language=en.

3. Orenstein, *Peggy. Girls & Sex: Navigating the Complicated New Landscape*, 72. New York: Harper, 2017.

4. Ibid.

5. Ibid, 71.

6. Simpson Rowe, Lorelei, Ernest N. Jouriles, Renee McDonald, Cora G. Platt, and Gabriella S. Gomez. "Enhancing Women's Resistance to Sexual Coercion: A Randomized Controlled Trial of the Date Program." *Journal of American College Health*60, no. 3 (2012): 211–18. https://doi.org/10.1080/07448481.2011.587068.

7. Tolman, Deborah L. *Dilemmas of Desire: Teenage Girls Talk about Sexuality*, 21. Cambridge: Harvard University Press, 2009.

8. Ibid.

9. Adichie, Chimamanda Ngozi. "*We Should All Be Feminists*". *TED Talks*, 2013. https://www.ted.com/talks/chimamanda_ngozi_adichie_we_should_all_be_feminists/up-next?language=en.

10. Orenstein, "What Young Women Believe about Their Own Sexual Pleasure."

11. Knapp, *Appetites*, 130.

12. Paquette, Danielle. "Why Frat Bros Can Throw Parties but Sorority Sisters Aren't Allowed To." *Washington Post*, April 29, 2019. https://www.washingtonpost.com/news/wonk/wp/2016/01/22/why-frats-can-throw-parties-but-sororities-cant/.

13. Pollack, Nicholas Russell. "Entitled Men and Guilty Women." *Chronicle*. Duke University, March 28, 2014. https://www.dukechronicle.com/article/2014/03/entitled-men-and-guilty-women.

14. Ibid.

15. Ibid.

16. Fulu, E., Warner, X., Miedema, S., et al. (2013). *Why Do Some Men Use Violence Against Women and How Can We Prevent It? Quantitative Findings from the United Nations Multi-country Study on Men and Violence in Asia and the Pacific.* Bangkok: UNDP, UNFPA, UN Women and UNV.

17. Glass, Gary. 'Sexual Entitlement on Campus."
18. Ibid.
19. Ibid.

Chapter 33

1. Engel, *Nice Girl Syndrome*, 15.
2. Ibid.
3. Ibid, 3.

Chapter 34

1. Rosin, Hanna. *The End of Men and the Rise of Women*, 22. London: Penguin, 2013.
2. Freitas, *End of Sex*, 11.
3. Glass, "Sexual Entitlement on Campus."
4. Vedantam, Shankar, Renee Klahr, Tara Boyle, Jennifer Schmidt, Rhaina Cohen, Maggie Penman, and Chloe Connelly. "Hookup Culture: The Unspoken Rules of Sex on College Campuses." NPR, February 14, 2017. https://www.npr.org/2017/02/14/514578429/hookup-culture-the-unspoken-rules-of-sex-on-college-campuses.

Chapter 35

1. Duke Student Broadcasting. "Me Too Monologues 2015: 'Girls' Night' & 'Looking.'" YouTube. February 19, 2015. Recorded theater performance, 9:24. https://www.youtube.com/watch?v=5k4k4rF-IFw.
2. Migdon, Brooke. "US LGBTQ+ Population Hits 20 Million." The Hill, December 14, 2021. https://thehill.com/changing-america/respect/diversity-inclusion/585711-us-lgbtq-population-hits-20-million.

3. Schmidt, Samantha. "1 In 6 Gen Z Adults Are LGBT. And This Number Could Continue to Grow." *The Washington Post*. WP Company, February 26, 2021. https://www.washingtonpost.com/dc-md-va/2021/02/24/gen-z-lgbt/.

4. *Violence and LGBTQ+ Communities: What Do We Know, and What Do We Need to Know?* Research Triangle Park: RTI International, 2017. https://www.rti.org/sites/default/files/rti_violence_and_lgbtq_communities.pdf. Accessed August 28, 2021.

5. Duke Student Broadcasting. "Lezbehonest—Lizzy Raben." YouTube. March 21, 2014. Recorded theater performance, 5:41. https://www.youtube.com/watch?v=pxZKYCe3W_Y.

6. Dionne, Evette. "Sorry Feminists, I'm Too Oppressed to Hook Up." *Mic*, July 30, 2013. https://mic.com/articles/57179/sorry-feminists-i-m-too-oppressed-to-hook-up#.kkF6wDljF.

7. Ibid.

8. Crenshaw, Kimberle. "Mapping the Margins: Intersectionality, Identity Politics, and Violence against Women of Color." *Stanford Law Review* 43, no. 6 (1991): 1241–99. https://doi.org/10.2307/1229039.

9. Hale, Chelsea, and Meghan Matt. "The Intersection of Race and Rape Viewed through the Prism of a Modern-Day Emmett Till." American Bar Association, July 16, 2019. https://www.americanbar.org/groups/litigation/committees/diversity-inclusion/articles/2019/summer2019-intersection-of-race-and-rape/.

Chapter 36

1. Reitman, "Sex & Scandal at Duke."

2. Lo, Rita. "Dating@Duke." Digital image. *Chronicle*, Duke University. September 30, 2015. Accessed February 2015.

3. Peterson, Cara. "The Farce of Duke's Hook-up Culture." *Chronicle*. Duke University, March 5, 2015. https://www.dukechronicle.com/article/2015/03/farce-dukes-hook-culture.

4. Asher, Steven R, and Molly Stroud Weeks. *Social Relationships, Academic Engagement, and Well-Being in College: Findings from the Duke Social Relationships Project*. Durham, NC: Duke University, 2015. http://www.dukechronicle.com/articles/2014/04/22/survey-highlights-campus-inequities-among-genders#.VPdCcpE0xCQ.

5. England, Paula, Emily Fitzgibbons Shafer, and Allison C.K. Fogarty. "Hooking Up and Forming Romantic Relationships on Today's College Campuses." *The Gendered Society Reader*, no. 5th (2012): 559–72. Oxford University Press.

6. Freitas, *End of Sex*, 35.

7. Glass, "Sexual Entitlement on Campus."

Chapter 37

1. Hinshaw, Stephen P., and Rachel Kranz. "Girls in Crisis." Introduction, *The Triple Bind: Saving Our Teenage Girls from Today's Pressures*. New York: Ballantine Books, 2009.

2. Hinshaw and Kranz, *Triple Bind*, 12.

3. Brown, *Gift of Imperfection*, 39.

4. Kross, E., M. G. Berman, W. Mischel, E. E. Smith, and T. D. Wager. "Social Rejection Shares Somatosensory Representations with Physical Pain." *Proceedings of the National Academy of Sciences* 108, no. 15 (2011): 6270–75. https://doi.org/10.1073/pnas.1102693108.

5. Brown, *Daring Greatly*, 232.

Chapter 38

1. Simmons, *Enough as She Is*, 45.

2. Ibid, 27.

3. Scelfo, Julie. "Suicide on Campus and the Pressure of Perfection." *New York Times*, July 27, 2015. https://www.nytimes.com/2015/08/02/education/edlife/stress-social-media-and-suicide-on-campus.html.

4. Fagan, Kate. "Split Image." ESPNW. ESPN Internet Ventures, May 7, 2015. http://www.espn.com/espn/feature/story/_/id/12833146/instagram-account-university-pennsylvania-runner-showed-only-part-story.

5. Frazee, Gretchen, and Patty Gorena Morales. "Suicide among Teens and Young Adults Reaches Highest Level since 2000." PBS, June 18, 2019. https://www.pbs.org/newshour/nation/suicide-among-teens-and-young-adults-reaches-highest-level-since-2000.

6. Piscopo, Kathryn Downey. "Suicidality and Death by Suicide Among Middle-Aged Adults in the United States." SAMHSA. https://www.samhsa.gov/data/sites/default/files/report_3370/ShortReport-3370.html. Accessed August 2, 2021.

7. Fagan, "Split Image."

Chapter 39

1. Denizet-lewis, Benoit. "Why Are More American Teenagers than Ever Suffering from Severe Anxiety?" *New York Times*, October 11, 2017. https://www.nytimes.com/2017/10/11/magazine/why-are-more-american-teenagers-than-ever-suffering-from-severe-anxiety.html.

2. "Mental Illness Prolific Among College Students." National Association of Mental Illness. https://www.nami.org/Press-Media/Press-Releases/2004/Mental-Illness-Prolific-Among-College-Students. Accessed August 29, 2021.

3. "Women's Increased Risk of Depression." Mayo Clinic. Mayo Foundation for Medical Education and Research, January 29, 2019. https://www.mayoclinic.org/diseases-conditions/depression/in-depth/depression/art-20047725.

4. Hinshaw and Kranz, *Triple Bind*, 31.

5. Ibid, 30.

6. Ibid, 32–36.

7. Glass, Gary. "Rethinking Campus Mental Health." *Inside Higher Ed*, May 29, 2019. https://www.insidehighered.com/views/2019/05/29/colleges-should-focus-more-community-and-connections-address-student-mental-health.

8. Rosin, Hanna. "The Silicon Valley Suicides." *Atlantic*, November 20, 2015. https://www.theatlantic.com/magazine/archive/2015/12/the-silicon-valley-suicides/413140/.

9. Fagan, Kate. *What Made Maddy Run: The Secret Struggles and Tragic Death of an All-American Teen*, 201–3. New York: Little, Brown and Company, 2018.

Chapter 40

1. Giwa-Osagie, Adesuwa. "Humans of Duke Facebook Post." Email, 2014.

2. Ibid.

3. Ward, Earlise C., Jacqueline C. Wiltshire, Michelle A. Detry, and Roger L. Brown. "African American Men and Women's Attitude toward Mental Illness, Perceptions of Stigma, and Preferred Coping Behaviors." *Nursing Research* 62, no. 3 (2013): 185–94. https://www.ncbi.nlm.nih.gov/pmc/articles/PMC4279858/.

4. Wong, Eunice C., Rebecca L. Collins, Jennifer Cerully, Rachana Seelam, and Beth Roth. "Racial and Ethnic Differences in Mental Illness Stigma and Discrimination among Californians Experiencing Mental Health Challenges." *Rand Health Quarterly* 6, no. 2 (January 13, 2017): 6. https://www.ncbi.nlm.nih.gov/pmc/articles/PMC5568160/.

Chapter 41

1. Ensler, Eve. *Insecure at Last: Losing It in Our Security-Obsessed World*, xiv–xv. New York: Villard, 2008.

2. Ibid, 72.

3. Ibid, xx.

4. Bowler, Kate. *Everything Happens for a Reason: And Other Lies I've Loved*, 26. New York: Random House, 2019.

5. Ibid, 119.

6. Glass, Gary. "PPT on Control." Email, 2015.

Chapter 42

1. Stossel, Scott. *My Age of Anxiety: Fear, Hope, Dread, and the Search for Peace of Mind*, 56. New York: Alfred A. Knopf, 2015.

2. Strayed, Cheryl. *Tiny Beautiful Things: Advice on Love and Life from Dear Sugar*, 287. New York: Vintage Books, 2012.

3. Rubin, Gretchen. *The Happiness Project*, 74. New York: HarperCollins Publishers, 2012.

4. Rilke, Rainer Maria. *Letters to a Young Poet.* Translated by Franz Xaver Kappus and Stephen Mitchell. Merchant Books, 2012.

Lastly, thank you to *Inside Higher Ed, The Week, Ms. Magazine, SheKnows Media, Rewire News, Elite Daily, Garnet News, Women's E-News, Bustle,* the National Eating Disorders Association, and the *Chronicle* for permission to use variations of articles I published with them in this book.

About the Author

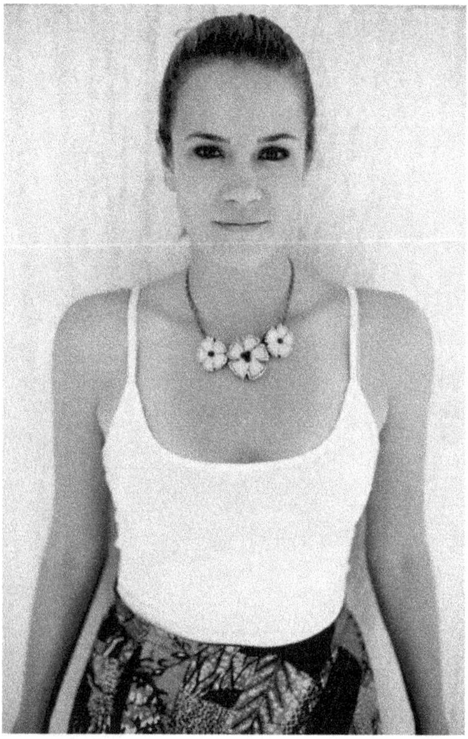

Caralena Peterson graduated from Duke University in 2015 with majors in Women's Studies and Public Policy. She has published articles with *Inside Higher Ed*, *The Week*, *She Knows Media*, *Ms. Magazine*, *Rewire News*, *Bustle*, *Garnet News*, and *Elite Daily*. She is also a mixed-medium artist whose work has appeared in the *New York Times* and *Washington Life Magazine*. When she is not busy with all her side hustles, Caralena works full-time as an English teacher in New Orleans, Louisiana.

To check out more of her work, to book her for a speaking gig, or to sign up for her newsletter, visit www.caralenapeterson.com. Keep your eyes peeled for an upcoming podcast!

CPSIA information can be obtained
at www.ICGtesting.com
Printed in the USA
BVHW041701220323
660957BV00010B/64/J

9 781633 376670